"There's perhaps no clearer testament to the man's ?
When you Google 'marathon training' or 'half ma......on training,'
Higdon's is the first name that you'll see."

—Runner's World, *October 2015.*
Hal Higdon listed as a Guru in the "50 Most Influential People in Running"

"I ran my first marathon 15 years ago and like nearly every first-time marathoner
I meet in my job, I used his marathon training plan. It is remarkable that no one
has dethroned Mr. Higdon from the top spot."

—*Chris Heuisler, Westin Hotel's national running concierge*

Praise for *Run Fast*, 1st edition

"Vintage Higdon. Hal brings perspective to his discussion and demonstrates
every point with a story out of his own experience or that of many other runners,
coaches, and scientists. A wealth of information."

—*David L. Costill, PhD, Ball State University*

"With *Run Fast*, Hal Higdon has put 'human' into the
science of human performance."

—*Russell R. Pate, PhD, University of South Carolina*

Praise for *Masters Running*

"Reaching 40 is not the end, but the beginning, for runners. In *Masters Running*,
Hal Higdon not only tells them how to stay fit and improve performance, he
inspires them to success."

—*David H. R. Pain, founder, masters movement*

"Hal Higdon has written the complete book of masters running. Nobody has done
it better. A very readable book, but also one that offers the advice that every
masters runner needs to know."

—*Al Sheahen,* National Masters News

"Clearly written, precisely focused, *Masters Running* is a typical Hal Higdon
work. It will make you the best age-group running that you can be."

—*Amby Burfoot, editor-at-large,* Runner's World *magazine*
and 1968 Boston Marathon champion

Also by Hal Higdon

On the Run from Dogs and People

The Electronic Olympics

Fitness After Forty

Beginner's Running Guide

Runner's Cookbook

The Marathoners

The Masters Running Guide

Marathon: The Ultimate Training Guide

Boston: A Century of Running

Hal Higdon's How to Train

Hal Higdon's Smart Running

Run, Dogs, Run!

Marathoning A to Z

Masters Running

Marathon: A Novel

Through the Woods

4:09:43: Boston 2013 Through the Eyes of the Runners

Hal Higdon's Half Marathon Training

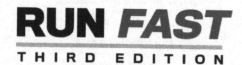

RUN *FAST*
THIRD EDITION

Completely Revised & Updated Third Edition

RUN FAST

How to Beat Your Best Time
EVERY TIME

HAL HIGDON

RODALE.

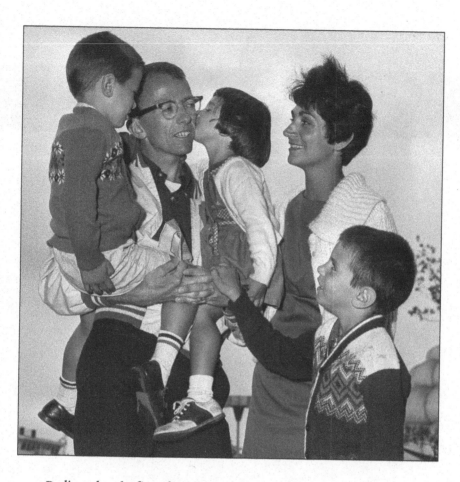

Dedicated to the five of us who were captured by a photographer for
The New York Times *after a race I won at the 1965 World's Fair—*
Rose and I and our three children: Kevin, David, and Laura.
Also dedicated to our nine grandchildren: Kyle, Wesley, Angela,
Holly, Jake, Nick, Sophie, David, and Danny.

Celebrating also the 50th anniversary of Runner's World
and the half century we have spent together.

—Hal Higdon

CONTENTS

INTRODUCTION
"If you want to run fast, you have to run fast." • xi

INTRODUCTION

"If you want to run fast, you have to run fast."

While writing the first edition of *Run Fast*, I talked to Lynn Jennings, who at the time was one of America's fastest female runners. Jennings won the IAAF World Cross Country Championships three times between 1990 and 1992, and placed third in the 10,000 at the 1992 Olympic Games in Barcelona. When considering the simple, two-word title of my book, Jennings commented: "If you want to run fast, you have to run fast."

There is a lot of truth to that remark, but if that was all that could be said about running fast, then you would not be holding this copy of a 200-plus page book in your hands. What made the first edition of *Run Fast*, published in 1992, and the second edition, published in 2000, bestsellers? Why am I able to boast that this third edition will enable you to improve as a runner at every distance from 5K to the marathon? Running fast is about more than heading out the door and simply picking up the pace of your daily workouts. The secret, as Jennings certainly knew, is achieving a balance of various elements that will ultimately teach you *how* to run fast, *when* to run fast, and *how much* "fast" running a structured program should include. What is my training program like if I'm a novice runner? What if I'm an experienced runner? Is there any room in a "fast" running program for "slow" running? Must a person's running life be dominated by speed-work day after grinding day? The answers to those training questions are at the heart and soul of this completely revised third edition of one of my most successful books.

So much has changed during the quarter century since the publication of the first edition of *Run Fast.* And yet so much remains the same. Humor me: Let's look backward to Training Past before we look forward to Training Future. To succeed in running during the final decade of the last century, elite athletes, Jennings's running peers, needed to run a lot of miles, most often in two-a-day workouts. Some of those miles could be slow (quantity counts), but many of those miles needed to be fast (quality counts even more). Speedwork a quarter century ago included interval training, repeats, sprints, strides, tempo runs, FCRs (fast continuous runs), and fartlek. I'll address each of those training methods later, but for now it's enough to know that all these pieces were on the chessboard back in the 1990s. Most experienced runners knew how to train way back when, and they succeeded by applying basic training methods that were disseminated widely, particularly in the pages of *Runner's World* magazine.

After reviewing the literature available today, examining the various books written in the last quarter century, but more important, talking to today's athletes and coaches, I'm not sure anyone has come up with a new form of speedwork. Certainly nothing new enough to hang a bestselling book on. In the first and second editions of *Run Fast,* I used "The Magic Workout" as the title for the chapter on interval training. As it turns out, it's still the magic workout today. Other than that, much has changed in the running sport. This third edition of *Run Fast* will address these changes.

RUNNING WILD

If anything has changed since the 1990s, it is the increase in the sheer number of runners participating in races that range in distance between 5K (3.1 miles) and the marathon (26.2 miles). Huge numbers. Numbers unimaginable when I wrote the first edition of this book. Running has exploded in popularity, as documented by Running USA, the statistical supersource for our sport. In its annual compilation of participant numbers, Running USA tells us that back in 1990, the number of people who finished half marathons was 303,000, and 224,000 finished full marathons. That seemed like a lot of runners back then, but those numbers increased exponentially to 1,986,600 and 509,000 respectively in 2015 (the most recent year for which statistics are available as I write this book).

Those two distances—the half marathon and the full marathon—garner a lot of attention from the statisticians as well as from the media and reporters like me. Visit your local bookstore or go online: Books about running crowd the shelves, in both print and electronic formats. Two of my running books are specific to those two distances, the full and the half marathon. But many more runners participate in 5K races: 8,300,000 in 2014, four times the number of those participating in the popular half marathon. The 5K also claims 44 percent of the finishers in all US running events. (Running USA counts only finishers, not entrants, when compiling numbers.) Another interesting statistic: A majority of those running 5K races are women (58 percent). Indeed, the ladies are driving the current and continuing boom in long-distance running.

Strikingly, the once top-ranked 10K (6.2 miles) attracts relatively fewer participants, at least as measured as a percentage of runners. Now the poor stepchild of the running boom, in 2015 the 10K attracted 1,275,660. But don't feel sorry for the 10K, because several of the highest profile road races are at that distance. Biggest is the Peachtree Road Race, held each Fourth of July in Atlanta. In 2015, 54,752 runners participated in that event. On Running USA's list of largest races, the New York City Marathon was the second largest with 49,365 that same year. Third and fourth were Bolder Boulder (a 10K in Colorado) with 45,336 runners and the Lilac Bloomsday Run (a 12K in Spokane, Washington) with 42,294. The Chicago Marathon filled out the top five with 37,395. Nobody can deny the popularity of distance running, whether shorter distances (5K and 10K) or longer distances (half and full marathons).

Some of those who participate in shorter distance events run them for fun, to fill time between half and full marathons. But probably a greater number of participants are perfectly content to do a local 5K or 10K now and then, with no desire to run farther or to run faster. I have to confess that after a long and successful career in open and master races, I share that level of contentment. With a smile on my face, I wander onto the course of short distance races well after the elites have taken off and join the walkers and joggers in the last starting grid. How many of those Peachtree runners, like me now, are indifferent to how fast they run? Certainly a few. But improvement does not always hinge on fast times, as recorded by your GPS watch or an app on your smartphone. Improvement comes in many packages, as you will learn in *Run Fast*. Would this book sell more copies if it were retitled *Run Comfortably*? No, but that is an important point. To see improvement, you must go beyond your comfort zone, either mentally or physically.

One factor that may hold many runners back when it comes to improving their time is the worry that if they push too hard, if they run too fast and too often, running will turn into a painful experience. They fear that running fast will increase their risk of injury. Certainly many new runners and even experienced runners equate running fast with pain. Running fast can both leave you out of breath and cause your muscles to ache after workouts. That may frighten many new runners, and experienced runners too may not want to get out of their comfort zone, at least not too often. Both groups may worry that by changing their training regimen to include fast running they are courting injury. "Speed kills," so we are warned.

Yet *Run Fast* never was intended to inflict pain. *Run Fast* in its various editions has not been merely about seeking personal records (PRs) at various race distances. Sure, we'd all like to return home from the local road race with a trophy in hand—but that's not the only reason we run. We like to feel good running. We like to look good running. We like to feel the wind in our hair. And yes, we'd all like to be able to run just a little faster—even if only to cut our 5K PR from 30:01 to 29:59.

HOW TO RUN FAST

Before you move from this introduction into the information-dense chapters, consider the science of *Run Fast*. Pay attention: It is a physiological fact that if you can run faster at shorter distances such as the 5K, you will be able to improve your performances at longer distances as well. All of your times will improve. "Speed is basic to performance at all levels," insists David L.

Costill, PhD. Check one of the performance charts or race predictors available on the Internet if you don't believe him. As the founder of the Human Performance Laboratory at Ball State University in Muncie, Indi-

Run faster at shorter distances such as the 5K, you will be able to improve your performances at longer distances as well.

ana, Dr. Costill is a leading expert in exercise physiology. If you can run a mile in 7:30, then—theoretically, at least—you should be able to do about 25:00 for a 5K, 52:00 for a 10K, 1:56 for the half marathon, and 4:00 for the full marathon.

But shave 15 seconds off that mile time and—again, theoretically—your times at longer distances should improve to about 24:30, 51:00, 1:54, and 3:55. Equally important, you'll feel better running. Your stride will feel smoother. You'll be able to converse while jogging, rather than gasping for breath with every step. Get in really good shape, and you'll recover more rapidly, which will allow you to run more often, or run longer distances, or have enough energy after your workout to want to go out dancing that evening. All sorts of good things will happen if you learn how to run fast. Of course, to do so, you'll need to teach yourself how to train for speed—which is what this book is all about.

While numerous books have shown people how to start jogging and how to finish their first marathon, less attention has been paid to running short races faster. Most runners will run a 5K as their first competitive experience. Others skip straight to the marathon, but eventually turn to 5K and 10K races because running road races is fun. You can't run marathons every weekend.

Unfortunately, few of the millions of people who are participating in the current running boom learned to run fast while they were younger. Most skipped high school track and cross-country, where they might have learned the skills necessary for successful running from an experienced coach. They did not run in college, either, except maybe recreationally. They never were coached as part of an athletic team. As a result, they missed the training opportunities at various levels when dedicated workouts with likeminded runners might have been available to help them. They never learned how to warm up properly. They never learned about interval training, fartlek, and bounding drills. "They never learned how to train for speed," explains Robert Vaughan, PhD, a coach in Dallas, Texas.

While researching the first edition of this book, I spoke with numerous world-class runners and their coaches. Talented and well-trained, these fast athletes often felt that the answers to my questions about improving speed were almost too simple. Having arrived at our sport via the traditional route, through high school and college competition to elite (professional) racing, they instinctively knew the type of training required to reach peak performance. And if they didn't know, they often had knowledgeable coaches who directed their training on a daily or even twice-daily basis. After years spent as highly competitive runners, they also understood that achieving top speed in a specific race required more than a few fast workouts. They knew it required a base of endurance before beginning those speed workouts. It required planning, organization, and a knowledge of other disciplines, from diet to strength to flexibility to racing tactics. It also required a lot of trial and error, since what works for others in training may not necessarily work for them. They knew it required body knowledge and body sensitivity. And even with all that in place, they knew achieving results still might require the assistance of an experienced coach.

At the time of the first edition of *Run Fast*, only the most gifted runners had access to first-class coaching: coaches in high school; coaches in college; coaches in clubs. However, over the last quarter century coaching has become increasingly available to runners at all levels. TrainingPeaks, the organization in Boulder, Colorado, that distributes my interactive training programs in daily e-mails to runners all over the world, provides a platform for several thousand coaches who in turn work one-on-one with runners at all levels. Never before has first-class coaching been so accessible to so many people. With this sort of support, athletic improvements are almost guaranteed.

All sorts of good things will happen if you learn how to run fast.

Let's hear it for our coaches. Hands together, everybody. They make us what we are. During my long running career, I have worked with numerous coaches and have learned something new from each of them. I also have had the opportunity to visit the laboratories of eminent exercise physiologists and physicians. They tested me on treadmills to increase their own knowledge, and in the bargain I usually went home a wiser runner.

As contributing editor for *Runner's World* magazine (my first article appeared in that publication's second issue back in 1966), I have shared information with millions of readers who run. In that position, I have had the opportunity to meet and interview many of the world's most knowledgeable coaches. Although their philosophies and training techniques often differed, these coaches shared a basic ability and desire to motivate athletes. They also knew how to teach athletes—some of them gifted, some of them less gifted—to reach for and achieve new goals.

Now it's time for you to reach for a new goal. You can improve as a runner at every distance, from the 5K to the marathon. You can run fast.

—*Hal Higdon*

Long Beach, Indiana

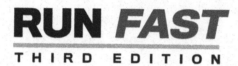

RUN *FAST*

THIRD EDITION

CHAPTER ONE

SECRETS OF SPEED

A dozen proven methods to make you a faster runner

Regardless of age or ability, almost all runners would like to improve. They would like to run faster. They would like to be able to run farther. They would like to maximize their talents. And, equally as important, they would like to make running easier and more fun regardless of time spent and distance covered.

Improvement: It's what we all desire.

Unfortunately, there is no magic formula, no kiss from a Prince Charming, that will turn a slow runner into a fast runner. Improvement does not come in a bottle. Wish-granting genies exist only in folktales and Disney movies. Becoming a faster runner takes hard work. It takes determination. It takes time; it takes not merely a few weeks or months to achieve a basic level of fitness, but a number of years. Perhaps most important, improvement needs a plan. Nevertheless, if you master the dozen or so secrets of speed I am about to offer in this chapter and the chapters that follow, you can improve as a runner. You can run fast.

While gathering information for this book, I did a survey online, asking runners who followed me on Facebook and Twitter to say what training methods worked best for them when it came to improvement. If they chopped a few seconds off their 5K time, if they sliced a few minutes off of their marathon time, what allowed that to happen? While I respect coaches and scientists and often use them as sources in my books and articles, lately I have begun to turn more and more to runners as my experts, because interpreting the results of laboratory experiments is not always easy. Connecting the dots, following the links from scientists through coaches and finally to runners, can be difficult at times. Also, not all runners have access to academic journals. Not all runners attend meetings of the American College of Sports Medicine. Not all runners even bother to read *Runner's World,* the bible of our sport. And even with the mass of information about long-distance running available in print and online, how do you apply it to you, the runner? What is the "you" factor when it comes to running fast?

Let me offer my approach: If you want to learn what works in this sport of ours, ask a runner.

In doing just that, I identified a dozen ways by which runners can improve, not only in competition, but in their ability to glide comfortably down the road during workouts. Few of us are athletically gifted enough to compete in an Olympic arena, but we all want to enjoy our sport and avoid the pitfalls of poor training, which often result in overuse injuries that keep us from running on a daily basis.

THE SECRETS OF SUCCESS

Very briefly, here is the list I came up with after I asked runners what worked for them when seeking to improve.

1. Running more miles
2. Training at a faster pace
3. Adding speedwork
4. Cross-training
5. Strength training
6. Stretching appropriately
7. Avoiding injuries
8. Following a good training program
9. Locating training partners
10. Joining a running club
11. Enlisting a coach
12. Training consistently, if not spectacularly

THE SECRETS OF SUCCESS

Sounds simple, doesn't it? Any one of you can apply any one of these suggestions and improve as a runner. Employ all of them, and you can improve even more. Let's quickly analyze each of these 12 elements to determine why they are the secrets to success.

1. **Running more miles.** This almost seems too obvious. Add a few miles to your daily and weekly running, and improvement will follow. All of my training programs embrace this philosophy and ask runners to gradually add miles as they progress from week to week. Jason Vallimont, 35, a science teacher from Grand Blanc, Michigan, agrees: "I improved by adding more miles, while at the same time avoiding injury by training at a slower pace."

2. **Training at a faster pace.** This seems to contradict the first piece of advice above, but even while adding miles you can still run some of those miles faster. Every workout should not be done at the same pace. On at least one day a week, run at race pace (race pace is the pace you plan to run in the race for which you are training). Doing so will help you to nail that same pace in competition.

3. **Adding speedwork.** Say "speedwork" and it scares many new runners. They fear the pain that supposedly accompanies grinding sessions on a track. Well, sometimes speedwork is painful. But speedwork does not need to be hard according to Nigel Grier from Dromore, Northern Ireland: "Put in most of your miles at an easy pace, which allows you to focus your attention on speedwork. This way you will improve without blasting every workout."

4. **Cross-training.** Adding or substituting other sports can help you maintain if not improve your aerobic fitness. Tim Lewis, 26, a sorter from Vinton, Virginia, did speed drills on a treadmill until it led to shin splints. "I shifted to the elliptical trainer, and it actually helped improve my speed."

5. **Strength training.** Strength equals speed. You need strength to succeed, particularly when the finish line is in sight and all systems used to
   propel you forward are about to break down. Ailéin Ó Clúmháin, 53, a
   teacher from Derry, Northern Ireland, says, "I felt like it gave me an
   extra gear, an added bonus over people whom I knew had not done any
   strength training."

6. **Stretching appropriately.** Scientists have a hard time proving that
   stretching can either prevent injuries or provide a means of rapid recovery. Nevertheless, most runners believe both be true. Hazel Wightman,
   48, an exercise physiologist from Harrisburg, Pennsylvania, states: "I
   have learned from personal experience that the most effective preventive for me is very gentle but regular stretching."

7. **Avoiding injuries.** Easier said than done, but injuries can be minimized,
   if not entirely avoided, if you pay attention to these other 11 tips. Is there
   one best way to avoid injuries? Listen to Megan Leahy, DPM, a Chicago
   podiatrist: "Investing the time into a gait analysis and running shoe fit-
   ting on the front end can hopefully keep you out of the podiatrist's office.
   Many of the injuries I see can be traced back to worn-out shoes or the
   wrong shoe for your foot type."

8. **Following a good training program.** Let me confess a certain bias
   when I offer advice on which program to use; after all, I promote training programs both on my Web site and through TrainingPeaks. Nevertheless, intelligent training rules every time. Nicolas Garcia, 40, a civil
   servant from London, England, agrees: "Learning how to put it all
   together and self-coach is the key."

9. **Locating training partners.** I now train mostly on my own for convenience, but for most of my career I partnered with runners near my ability
   for tough workouts on the track or long runs on the roads and in the
   woods. Tim Guimond, 62, an economic consultant from Evanston, Illinois, says, "I lowered my marathon time by 14 minutes and qualified for
   Boston after running with slightly faster runners."

10. **Joining a running club.** The best way to find running partners is by
    joining a club. The Road Runners Club of America contains 1,100 member

clubs, with 250,000 individual members. Clubs range in size from the Anniston (Alabama) Runners club with 350 members to the New York Road Runners with 40,000 members. "I ran my first road race hosted by Anniston when I was 10 years old," Jean Knaack, executive director of the RRCA, remembers fondly.

11. **Enlisting a coach.** Yes, coaches cost money, but it could be money well spent if it allows you to improve as a runner. Coach Roy Benson of Amelia Island, Florida, recommends: "Hire a coach with lots of experience who can practice the art as well as science of coaching. Experienced coaches have learned how to dig deeply into your background and current situation in order to develop a completely individualized training plan with workouts based on your history, current level of fitness, general ability, and both short- and long-term goals."

12. **Training consistently, if not spectacularly.** This might be the most important secret of all. Train at a comfortable level for a long time and tweak your training program from time to time, and you can *continue* to run fast. Cyndi Keough Springford, 43, a personal trainer from Plaistow, New Hampshire, says, "I firmly believe that consistency breeds competency and competency breeds confidence. You have to put the time in. You have to show up. Repetition is the mother of all skills."

Thank you to all the runners and experts who have helped me come up with these 12 secrets of success. But we're just getting started. These 12 secrets only hint at the depth of material available in the pages of *Run Fast*. Keep reading!

CHAPTER TWO

FLYING WITHOUT WINGS
The thrill of running fast

The feel of the wind in your hair. That's the best way I can describe running fast. Doing it provides almost a sensual pleasure. Simply stated, running fast feels good. It doesn't happen in every workout, or in every race, but on those special occasions when you're rested and eager and ready to run and you've found a perfect course featuring breathtaking scenery or you have a pleasant running partner, nothing could be better. Our urge to run fast is what pushes a lot of us out the door and down the road or onto a winding forest path each day. We like running, and we especially like running fast.

Some people equate this to achieving a "runner's high." Scientists suggest that at certain stress levels the body releases endorphins that find their way to our brains. *Wheee!* Feels good. A natural high. Who needs drugs, when you can go for a 40-minute tempo run down the road and suddenly feel like you're up in the air? Some claim they achieve this runner's high at least occasionally. Others say they never have experienced a runner's high, although maybe they just failed to recognize it. Regardless, running fast provides its own pleasure.

Julie Isphording, an Olympic marathoner and director of the Thanksgiving Race in Cincinnati sums it up. She says, "When you're running fast, it's pure joy. It's the exhilarating moment—the moment when you are breezing by the world. It's hot-blooded ecstasy, soaring intensity, when you can't feel the pavement, you can't hear your heart pounding, and you're flying without wings."

Who needs drugs, when you can go for a 40-minute tempo run down the road and suddenly feel like you're up in the air?

If you never have run before, it may be too early to suggest that someday you might be able to go airborne. Even if you are an experienced runner who has logged dozens of 5K and 10K races, it may take a while before you are willing to believe the message that you can improve as a runner. Can anybody be taught to run fast? I think they can.

Fast, of course, is a relative term. Fast for one runner is slow for another—and vice versa. On several occasions, I have competed in the Vulcan Run, a 10K in Birmingham, Alabama. On my first visit, when I was still in my 50s (a relative youngster), I ran the distance in about 35 minutes. On my second trip 15 years later, I competed in an accompanying 5K, running slower than 25 minutes. Speaking at the postrace dinner, I joked to the audience, "As I age, my times for the 5K have begun to approach my former times for the 10K."

But it didn't really matter. I felt fast on both occasions. You should have seen me coming down the final straightaway of the 5K: I was flying! Toward the end of his racing career, Jack Foster, the New Zealand Olympian, commented, "I feel like I'm running as fast as always—as long as I don't look at my watch." You might not be able to run 30 minutes for a 5K, or 60 minutes for a 10K, but no matter the distance you can still feel fast doing so.

Running fast does not take special talent. You don't need expensive equipment. You don't need to hire a coach or train on a track—although good coaching certainly can help, and tracks are where a lot of fast runners do hang out. Some skills are required, but the average runner can learn those skills. You don't need to participate in 5K and 10K races every weekend, although many runners enjoy a full racing schedule. Running fast requires mainly a change of attitude and a willingness to experiment with different workouts and training methods.

If you're a beginner, running fast means merely getting started. Any pace at all, no matter how slow, still beats sitting on the couch, drinking beer, and watching TV. If you've never exercised before, your first walk or run earns you a PR. If you've never run before, except when you were a child (when running was perceived as fun and not as hard work), your first few jogging steps will allow you to experience your youth again. Jogging for a few hundred meters is to move faster than if you were to walk that same distance. Improvement comes rapidly—if not always easily—when you begin from a base of zero fitness.

Fast for one runner is slow for another—and vice versa.

GETTING STARTED

Consider, for a moment, beginners who have not yet run their first 5K, much less begun to worry about running that distance even faster. If you are an experienced runner who bought this book to help you set a PR or qualify for the Boston Marathon, you may want to skip over to the next chapter. On the other hand, why not hang close? You never know when you might pick up a tip or two that will aid you as a runner.

The best advice anyone can offer a beginner is: Just do it! Begin easily. Take a few fast steps forward. Walk and jog without worrying whether there is anybody looking over your shoulder. Don't be shy. Don't be embarrassed. Stride forth with purpose. Anybody looking at you—specifically non-runners—probably do so in envy. Not everybody has the courage to begin. John Bingham, a *Runner's World* columnist and author of *Running for Mortals* (among his many books), frequently told audiences: "The miracle isn't that I finished. The miracle is that I had the courage to start."

In the words of Olympian Priscilla Welch, "If you want to become the best runner you can be, start now. Don't spend the rest of your life wondering if you can do it." Of course, Welch also knows it's never too late to start. A former heavy smoker, she did not even begin competitive running until she was in her mid-thirties—but she went on to make the British Olympic team and win the New York City Marathon.

Beginners occupy a unique—and fortunate—position in the running world because their every move is upward. "One of the joys of being a beginning runner is that you continue to get better," says Mary Reed of the Atlanta Track Club. "Everything is improvement until you reach that first plateau. It's an innocent time of joy in any runner's life that a lot of us would like to go back to."

> *"If you want to become the best runner you can be, start now."*

How do you begin? The answer to that question is both simple and complicated. Let's start by talking about motivation.

One winter night some years ago, I was changing in the locker room of the local racket club near where I live in Northwest Indiana when a tennis enthusiast inquired about the group of people nearby who were buzzing around me. "What are you doing?" he asked.

I explained about the beginning running class I was then teaching with my wife, Rose. At that time, we met with the group once a week to run together around the racket club's indoor track.

The tennis player seemed surprised: "I didn't know you could teach running."

He was right, of course. You don't need to teach running—or shouldn't need to. Children learn to run almost as soon as they learn to walk. Visit any elementary school playground, and you'll see kids running all over the place. An athlete who goes out for any sport in high school—football, basketball, tennis—runs as part of the conditioning program for that sport, or should! It is only as adults that people forget to run and sometimes have to "relearn" the motion. (One of my favorite T-shirt mottos, seen often at cross-country meets, is, "My sport is your sport's punishment.")

Running is basically a simple movement. Olympian Don Kardong, director of the Lilac Bloomsday Run, breaks the running movement into its simplest level: "You start out with either your left or right foot, and alternate." It's that simple.

When Rose and I taught people to run, we tried to get them to start slowly. Some beginners (particularly if they're overweight) need to walk first, beginning with a half hour, 3 or 4 days a week. We suggested that they jog a short distance until they got slightly out of breath, walk to recover, then jog some more. Jog, walk. Jog, walk. While Kardong's comment about putting your left or right foot forward is always good for a laugh when told at seminars, the truth is he precisely nails how beginners start to run.

Jog, walk. Jog, walk. It doesn't get much simpler than that. I don't need to write you a program. Cover whatever distance you comfortably can cover. After a few weeks, as you gradually begin to get in shape, you will find that you are able to jog for longer periods of time with shorter walking breaks in between. Eventually you should be able to run nonstop without walking breaks, although I'm not sure that end goal serves as a necessity anymore. Case in point is the success my fellow coach and running guru Jeff Galloway has had in teaching people to run marathons. He advises that individuals run with the intent to take regular walking breaks, sometimes spaced only a minute apart. ("Gallowalks," they sometimes are called.) Jeff estimates that, directly and indirectly and over a period of several decades, he has taught this method to as many as 400,000 runners/walkers. Beginners might do 5 to 10 seconds of easy jogging, walking the rest of the minute, for 10 to 12 minutes. More experienced runners might alternate between 4 minutes running and 30 seconds walking, moving at an 8:00 mile pace.

Interestingly, the jog-walk-jog-walk approach used by beginners mimics interval training, a very sophisticated method for improving racing performance. I'll cover interval training in detail in Chapter 13.

PREACHING MODERATION

When we taught beginners, we preached moderation, following the motto coined by New Zealand coach Arthur Lydiard: "Train, don't strain." We also talked about efficient running form, diet, equipment, safety, and avoiding injuries. Every now and then we showed a film featuring a running guru, such as Ken Cooper, MD, or the late George Sheehan, MD.

But mostly, we did not teach running; rather, we peddled motivation. Every coach of a beginning running class does the same. A lot of us who have been running more than a few years forget, but Bingham was right: It does take courage to don a pair of running shoes and step out on a sidewalk for the first time, in front of friends and neighbors. Quite honestly, a lot of beginning runners never get beyond the fear of looking foolish. They lack self-confidence. They fear failure.

One advantage of a class situation, of course, is the group support you get from others of similar ability. This certainly was true with the marathon class I helped supervise for many years in Chicago to prepare runners for that city's marathon. In the class, which was organized by the Chicago Area Runners Association (CARA), we usually had several thousand runners each summer. Certainly, everyone in the CARA class ran to the Kardongian right-foot-left-foot mantra.

But motivation is not only necessary for beginners. Motivation is the staple component at every level, from novice to expert. One reason why the East Africans have been able to dominate the world distance running ranks is that they train together and push each other every day in practice. Top runners gather in cities such as Eugene, Oregon, or Boulder, Colorado, for mutual support. Group dynamics can be very important in achieving success. If you have the opportunity to join a class or hire a coach or train with other runners, do so. You'll greatly increase your chances to run better—and faster!

CHAPTER THREE

BEGINNER'S LUCK

*You can't run fast unless
you first start to run*

When cold winds blow, when leaves drop from the trees, when frost covers the lawns, I know the time has come for my wife and me to follow the migrating birds southward to our second home in Florida. Rose and I winter in Ponte Vedra Beach, on the Atlantic Ocean just outside Jacksonville. At low tide, the beach offers a surf-battered surface: flat, smooth, springy—ideal for aging legs. The beach wills me to run fast.

One of our best Florida friends is Mary Ellen Reed. She lives only a few doors away in our condo complex, and we see her often. Each weekday Rose and Mary Ellen participate in a morning water aerobics class at a nearby fitness center. Recently, we began to notice that Mary Ellen often went for afternoon walks through the neighborhood or on the beach, probably a mile or two judging from the time it took her.

The number-one race in Jacksonville is the Gate River Run, a looping 15K (9.3 miles) that crosses two bridges over the St. Johns River near downtown. In addition to the 15K, there is also a 5K, untimed and with no awards other than the obligatory race T-shirt. Race director Doug Alred provides this satellite race more for joggers and walkers than hard-core runners. Sometimes I run the 15K, sometimes the 5K.

Rose asked Mary Ellen if she would like to do the 5K. Mary Ellen's immediate reaction was that she would never do a "race." Rose countered by telling Mary Ellen that she covered nearly that distance during her regular walks. Long story short, the three of us went to the Gate River Run. While I, heroically, did the 15K along with nearly 20,000 other runners, the two of them, also heroically, did the 5K. That course followed an easy out-and-back route through downtown Jacksonville. Because Mary Ellen had once lived in that area, she spent most of the "race" pointing out this church and that church among various other landmarks. Afterward, she proudly told us, "Now I can wear a race T-shirt."

It is often that simple. Big and small 5K races are everywhere: 16,100 of them in 2015, according to Running USA. Most reasonably fit people can walk, if not run, that distance without much training. At the same time, they can achieve greater success (run or walk faster) if they participate in a running class or use a training program.

FIRST-TIME RUNNING

I love hearing runners tell me about their first time running. Traci Dutko Strungis, 46, a registered nurse from Mountaintop, Pennsylvania, had parents who were runners. She ran cross-country in high school, though not seriously, she admits. But she knew the value of staying fit. "When I was in my late 20s I moved to Philadelphia. After mastering a step aerobics class, I felt I needed something more challenging, so I decided to try running again."

For her first run, Strungis chose the bike path on Kelly Drive, near the Philadelphia Museum of Art, whose 72 steps became famous after Sylvester Stallone ran up them in the film *Rocky*. Strungis's first run was 5 minutes out, then 5 minutes back. A guy on rollerblades had been watching and shouted, "Is that as far as you're going?"

She shouted back, "It's my first time running!"

"Now I can wear a race T-shirt."

Touché, rollerblader! Strungis, 6 months later, ran her first 5K. She would go on to run 22 marathons, including Boston, and serve on the board of directors of her local running club, the Wyoming Valley Striders.

David Allen, 48, a geologist from Houston, Texas, began running with his older brother after graduating from high school. They were on vacation in northern Wisconsin. "We went for a run on a quiet country road through the woods. I remember how good it felt to explore nature on foot, watching it pass with each new step. I also enjoyed the feeling of breathing hard, yet we ran slowly enough so I didn't get exhausted. We ran 2 miles, which at the time seemed like a major feat to me."

Yet two decades would pass before he ran his first half marathon and full marathon. "Even now when I run," Allen says, "I still enjoy that initial feeling of watching the world pass by with each step."

Hazel Wightman, 48, an exercise physiologist from Harrisburg, Pennsylvania, started at an age much younger than most runners. She was 4 years old when her family moved to a new house in Pittsburgh. The house was halfway up a big hill. "I asked my father if I could run to the top of the hill. He said no."

Stubbornly, the little 4-year-old asked again, "Do you mean I am not allowed to run to the top of the hill, or I am not able?"

Her father indicated the latter.

The next day, she tried—and failed. She tried again—and failed again. "I tried over and over," she says. "I did that day after day until I was able to run all the way to the top of the hill and show my dad that I could do it." Decades later, Wightman remains a runner.

Marc Wolfson, 65, retired and living in Olney, Maryland, was working at the United States Coast Guard headquarters in Washington, DC, when he quit smoking. Good choice, except it caused Wolfson to gain weight. He started working out at his office's exercise facility, which had a banked track on the roof, 17 laps to the mile. "They gave you a clicker to keep track of laps," recalls Wolfson. "I started with a mile and worked myself up to 3 miles on that little track, wearing a pair of blue-tipped Converse tennis shoes.

"Every time I ran, I could feel my lungs working. I traded a negative addiction for a positive addiction." Forty-two years later, Wolfson is still running.

LOOKING GOOD

For beginners, such as our friend Mary Ellen and the other first-timers, the most important thing a coach can tell them is not how to hold their arms or how far to jog without stopping or which one of Hal Higdon's training programs to follow. A coach simply needs to say, "You're looking good. You're doing great. Keep it up." Basic motivation is all these new runners need. Natural running instincts, developed in childhood, simply take over.

Regardless of whether your goal is a 5K or a marathon, finding a good running class is an important first step. Or a good coach. Jean Knaack, executive director of the Road Runners Club of America, tells me that the RRCA has certified more than 4,000 distance running coaches. They are located throughout the United States. "Our coaches work with runners in their running clubs and coach privately in small groups at one-on-one settings."

Many major road races provide classes for beginners, as well as for those planning to run their race. Simply check the race Web site to see if a class is offered. To find classes in your area, contact local running stores or fitness centers. Hospitals often offer "wellness programs." Or, try surfing the Internet. Also, community colleges often host classes in fitness, walking, jogging, and even marathon running. Running clubs usually welcome beginning joggers. Some, such as the Chicago Area Runners Association (CARA), Atlanta Track Club, and New York Road Runners Club (NYRR), offer personalized coaching. In addition to regular running classes, runners clubs such as NYRR offer treadmill classes, deep water classes, and yoga for runners. The NYRR's Bob Glover, author of *The Runner's Handbook*, estimates that along with his wife, Shelly, he has coached 100,000 runners, from first-time 5K runners to Olympic Marathon Trials qualifiers. "Our focus always has been on improving performance, no matter what level the runner's talent or experience."

Atlanta offers classes at all levels—beginners to marathon runners—with nearly 2,000 participants a year, according to coach Amy Begley, who ran the 10,000 meters race at the 2008 Olympic Games. In Chicago, CARA each year enrolls more than 2,000 participants in its marathon training programs (using my training plans), and also offers an "Intro to Running" class, focusing on the basics. In serving runners, CARA utilizes as many as 10 coaches and 400 volunteers.

To locate a running club in your area (or out-of-town clubs when traveling), check the RRCA's Web site (rrca.org). This is one easy way to plug into a network of runners; you'll be surprised how eager other runners and running clubs are to assist novice runners who are seeking advice and help.

TRAINING TERMS

The terms used in the training programs in this book are somewhat obvious, but clear-cut definitions never hurt.

■ **Rest:** Rest days are as important as training days. They give your muscles time to recover so you can run again. Actually, your muscles will build in strength as you rest. Without recovery days, you will not improve.

■ **Run:** Put one foot in front of the other and run. It sounds pretty simple, and it is. Don't worry about how fast you run or whether you have perfect running form; just cover the distance— or approximately the distance—suggested. Ideally, you should be able to run at a pace that allows you to converse comfortably while you do so.

■ **Walk/Run:** This is a combination of running and walking, suggested for those in-between days when you want to do some running, but only some. There is nothing in the rules that suggests you have to run continuously, either in training or in any races you choose to run later. Use your own judgment. Another option for in-between days is to cross-train: bike, swim, or simply walk.

■ **Walk:** Walking is an excellent exercise that a lot of runners overlook in their training. In the training schedule offered in this chapter, I suggest that you go for a walk measured in minutes rather than miles on the day after your longest run. Don't worry about how fast you walk, or how much distance you cover. Not all training should be difficult. A hike in a natural setting can add a little adventure to your walking routine.

TRAINING FOR BASE FITNESS

But in all honesty, do you need a coach or a running class to begin as a runner? Probably not. After all, running is such a simple activity, a one-step-at-a-time sport. Whether or not you eventually decide to seek outside support, you can begin on your own. For some people, it is even advisable that they begin on their own until they establish a basic level of fitness. In other words, first get in shape, then join a class that teaches you how to get in even better shape. So, before we move on to the subject of running faster, let's address the subject of running at any speed, your speed.

A simple 8-week training program can get you out the door or up onto the treadmill. Before you embark on the schedule, it is assumed that you have no major health problems, are in reasonably good shape, and have done at least some jogging or walking. If running a mile-and-a-half, as you will be asked to do at the end of the first week, seems too difficult, then you may want to schedule more than 8 weeks to reach your goal. Moreover, you might begin by walking, rather than running.

All of my training programs, including those for race distances that may not interest you at this point, follow a basic pattern from day to day and week to week. Let me start by explaining that pattern. Even if you are an experienced runner looking for advice on how to fine-tune your already remarkable training regimen, you need to pay attention.

Monday: Almost all of my programs schedule rest on Mondays. Taking a day off allows you to recover from any hard training you might have done over the weekend. Even the advanced programs for those who train 7 days a week recommend comparative rest: both fewer and slower miles.

Tuesday: Today you run. At the beginning of this program, you do not run very far: only a quarter mile. Review the "first-time" stories of some of the people mentioned in this chapter, and recall that they often struggled to get this far in their early workouts. Don't be too hard on yourself and do too much too soon.

Wednesday: An option day, depending on how Tuesday went. You can rest. You can walk. You can run. Speaking to the large number of readers of this book, I can't predict what might be best to you. But I trust you to listen to your body and make the right decision.

Thursday: Another running day, a mirror image of Tuesday. This program begins with a quarter-mile run. At the end of the program, after 8 weeks, you will reach a peak of 2 miles on Tuesdays and Thursdays.

Friday: More rest. Even in my most difficult and advanced training programs I want runners to rest. You can't train properly if you are not well rested. Rest is particularly important leading into the weekends, because that is where I prescribe the toughest training.

Saturday: Were the 5 previous days too easy? I usually make up for it on the weekends, when people have both more time and more energy to train hard. Can you call a 1.5-mile run in the first week a "long run"? It is for beginners. Over a period of 8 weeks, you will increase the distance a quarter-mile each week, peaking at 3 miles in Week 8.

Sunday: Go for a walk. I don't particularly care how fast, whether a stroll in the park or a power walk. Forget distance; use time for a barometer. Begin in Week 1 by walking for 25 minutes. Adding 5 minutes a week allows you to reach a full hour by Week 8.

Training programs are not about absolutes, they are about progression. And that is an important point: All of my training programs, and the training programs of almost all coaches who work with both beginning and experienced runners, are progressive. You start at an easy level; you progress to a harder level. You start with a short distance; you progress to a long distance. You start running slow; you progress to the point where you can run fast.

The pattern you see in this beginner training program essentially mirrors every training program I have developed—and I have more than

You start at an easy level;
you progress to a harder level.

60 such programs available online. If you check the training programs of other respected coaches, you will find that they also progress from one week to the next. Why? Because it works. Training progressively harder over a period of weeks and months and years allows you to become a faster runner. That is, if you don't pick too steep a ramp for your progression. Hopefully, by the time you finish reading this book, you will have figured out how to do just that.

A BASIC BEGINNING: 1

Here is your first training program. If you feel this is way too easy for you, if you have been running for years and competing in races from 5K to the marathon, skip ahead. If I have insulted you by suggesting that you might have difficulty running only a quarter mile on your Tuesday and Thursday workouts, oh well. You'll get over it, particularly as you develop your ability to run fast.

Want to run precisely a quarter mile (0.25 mile) or a half mile (0.5 mile) or

A Basic Beginning: 1

WEEK	MON	TUE	WED	THU	FRI	SAT	SUN
1	Rest	0.25 mile run	Rest or run/walk	0.25 mile run	Rest	1.5 mile run	25 min walk
2	Rest	0.5 mile run	Rest or run/walk	0.5 mile run	Rest	1.75 mile run	30 min walk
3	Rest	0.75 mile run	Rest or run/walk	0.75 mile run	Rest	2.0 mile run	35 min walk
4	Rest	1.0 mile run	Rest or run/walk	1.0 mile run	Rest	2.25 mile run	40 min walk
5	Rest	1.25 mile run	Rest or run/walk	1.25 mile run	Rest	2.5 mile run	45 min walk
6	Rest	1.5 mile run	Rest or run/walk	1.5 mile run	Rest	2.75 mile run	50 min walk
7	Rest	1.75 mile run	Rest or run/walk	1.75 mile run	Rest	3.0 mile run	55 min walk
8	Rest	2.0 mile run	Rest or run/walk	2.0 mile run	Rest	3.0 mile run	60 min walk

more? There is an easy way to do it. Go to a running track. Most outdoor running tracks are exactly 400 meters long, which is just short of 440 yards, a quarter mile. If you run or walk in the inside lane, like you were competing in the Olympics, you can precisely measure the distance covered. At some tracks, however, slow runners and walkers are asked to exercise in the outside lanes. This may force you to adjust your distances somewhat, but don't worry about it. A lap is a lap, whether it is 400 meters, 440 yards, or farther than that.

A BASIC BEGINNING: 2

Here is a variation of the same training program. The only difference is that A Basic Beginning: 2 is based on time, while A Basic Beginning: 1 is based on distance. Simply, I converted the mileage numbers to minutes. You don't need to worry whether you have run a quarter mile or a mile or two miles. You may not have access to a precisely measured course like a track, and if you are a new runner you may not have a GPS watch to measure your mileage. And, quite honestly, the numbers you see on the screens of treadmills are not always accurate.

A Basic Beginning: 2

WEEK	MON	TUE	WED	THU	FRI	SAT	SUN
1	Rest	3 min run	Rest or run/walk	3 min run	Rest	18 min run	25 min walk
2	Rest	6 min run	Rest or run/walk	6 min run	Rest	21 min run	30 min walk
3	Rest	9 min run	Rest or run/walk	9 min run	Rest	24 min run	35 min walk
4	Rest	12 min run	Rest or run/walk	12 min run	Rest	27 min run	40 min walk
5	Rest	15 min run	Rest or run/walk	15 min run	Rest	30 min run	45 min walk
6	Rest	18 min run	Rest or run/walk	18 min run	Rest	33 min run	50 min walk
7	Rest	21 min run	Rest or run/walk	21 min run	Rest	36 min run	55 min walk
8	Rest	24 min run	Rest or run/walk	24 min run	Rest	36 min run	60 min walk

I'm going to assume that, as a beginner, you can run at a pace of 12 minutes a mile. If you run (or walk) slower or faster, feel free to make any needed adjustments to the schedule yourself.

These training program schedules are only guides. Feel free to make minor modifications to suit the weather and your work and family schedule.

MY VERY FIRST TIME

Most of the following individuals caught on quickly. Like them, start by running a little, then run a little bit more, and one day you'll realize you are a runner. In their own words:

Anna Weber, Michigan City, Indiana: I went out for cross-country in sixth grade thinking I had to carbo-load, because my mom told me that's what runners do. Before the first practice, I gobbled down a half-dozen pancakes. At 2 miles I puked up everything.

Lynn Lubbe, Burlington Township, New Jersey: Soon after meeting my future husband, I attempted to run with him. My running gear was all wrong. My stride and breathing were amateur. Dave never gave up on me, and our running has endured through two decades.

Connie Ciampanelli, North Providence, Rhode Island: The assignment for my first run was to go 60 seconds. I thought I would have to be scraped from the gutter. But soon I successfully completed a 5K.

Marisa Sauceda Jimenez, San Antonio, Texas: After walking on a treadmill and losing 50 pounds, I decided to try running outdoors. I came home drenched in sweat, and my husband asked what happened. I burst into tears and said, "I did it! I did it!"

Paula Hartson: I put my baby in his stroller for our first run. I only passed a single house before starting to walk for three or four houses. Every day, I would run a little farther and walk a little less. Then one day I completed a full mile without stopping. I knew then I could do it.

Most important, follow a progression that allows you to gradually improve your fitness level and ability to run farther more so than faster. There will be plenty of time to improve your speed as you continue to learn the tricks of the running trade.

Angelia Freeman, Roseburg, Oregon: Within seconds, everything hurt. My legs had no strength. My lungs couldn't figure out what was wrong, and my belly jiggled like piglets in a gunny-sack. I began to sweat. It was rolling off me in sheets, stinging my eyes, dripping off my elbows, I was slimy all over. It took me 4 months of treadmill running before I would go outside where people could see me.

Debbie Manser Martinez: My initial goal was to jog to a street light, walk to the next. Over and over. I ran my first half marathon 4 months later. It's still a love/hate relationship at times, but running has become my passion.

Erin Lynn, Shelbyville, Kentucky: I remember making little goals for myself, like run to this mailbox, take a walking break, then run to that light pole, etc. I remember the joy I felt when I didn't need that walk break.

Diane Howard, Staten Island, New York: My sixth-grade teacher started a club after school. I learned about endurance, stress relief, and the beauty of the running community. I will always be grateful to that sixth-grade teacher.

Sherry King, Baltimore, Maryland: I decided to go for a run with a friend. She would not stop talking the whole time. All I wanted to do was get it over with. But that day I fell in love with running. She remains my very best friend. Together we have run countless miles.

CHAPTER FOUR

GOING TO THE RACES: 5K NOVICE

Run 3 miles? You can do it

I t's a small race in a small town. Every Fourth of July, my family in Indiana organizes a 5K race at the Old School Community Center in the town of Long Beach. In earlier years, when we first moved to town, the sprawling one-story building housed the Long Beach School, unique in that it was designed by John Lloyd Wright, son of famed architect Frank Lloyd Wright, a former resident of our town on the shores of Lake Michigan. My wife, Rose, taught at that school.

Every Fourth of July, a hundred or more mostly local runners appear clasping $5 in their hands, which is all we charge for entry to the Old School Run, the money serving as a donation to the community center. Last year, with my granddaughter Holly serving as the race director, we raised more than $700.

Don't tell anybody, but the course is short. Maybe as much as a quarter-mile short. Guaranteed PR for 5K, provided you don't inquire too closely on the course's accuracy. No race numbers. No electronic timing. No places recorded. No age-group awards, but you are required to take home an old T-shirt, which is how the Higdon family cleans out its closets.

It is a scenic course that loops around a pond, woods, and nice homes.

Finishers get a bottle of water and a race certificate. The Old School Run is all about friends and family. As runners continue to finish, everyone stands around chatting: who just had a baby, who just graduated from school, who just got a new job, who just ran a marathon or a real race where they do have electronic timing. Then, as though someone blew a whistle signifying the fun is over, everyone disappears, heading home with plans to return to the park later for bratwurst, beer, and a parade.

It's the way running should be.

But the Thanksgiving Day Race in Cincinnati, Ohio, is also the way running should be. It is a 10K, twice the length of the Old School Run, and I can assure you that the race director, Julie Isphording, an Olympian, and a friend of mine for years, has had the course precisely measured and certified as accurate. Approximately 16,000 runners do the Thanksgiving Day Race each year, paying $35 for entry. This is actually quite a reasonable fee given today's market, where entry fees can reach $250 to $500 for major marathons.

The Thanksgiving Day Race is not the largest 10K in the United States. (That honor goes to the Peachtree Road Race, held on the Fourth of July in Atlanta, Georgia.) But, founded in 1908, it is among the oldest—*the* oldest being the Bemis-Forslund Pie Race (4.5 miles) in Gill, Massachusetts, founded in 1891. Worldwide, according to the Association of Road Race Statisticians, the Palio del Drappo Verde Half Marathon in Verona, Italy, traces its roots to the year 1208 (!), but it has not been run continuously since that date. The Thanksgiving Day Race attracted only 18 competitors its first year, missed a year in 1918 because of World War I, and missed another year in 1936 during the middle of the Great Depression. Nevertheless, the Cincinnati race possesses a gravitas that most race directors can only envy. "If you're looking for a slice of tradition to go with your turkey and pumpkin pie, running 10K on Thanksgiving in Cincinnati is the way to go," laughs Isphording. "The holiday tradition in Cincinnati centers around a 10K run on a really cold day with the whole family. No one questions it." As an aside, runners also contribute money to a dozen charities and donate an average of 10,000 pounds of clothing to an annual Goodwill clothing drive.

Whether they choose events large or small, runners love to race. People run for various reasons, but at least once a year many runners select a specific race to serve as focus for their training. It can be a local hometown fun run like the Old School Run or something a bit more serious. Just as there are numerous types of runners, there are countless races to choose from. Simply select a race that works for you.

For instance, Jason Coleman found himself 5 months into a new weight loss program. He was getting bored doing the elliptical every day.

"Running changed my life."

"I wanted more variety," says Coleman, who decided to take some of his workouts outdoors, beginning with a short walk and jog on a nearby street. An easy beginning with a door opening to a new lifestyle.

Being a fan of Walt Disney, Coleman chose a 10K at Walt Disney World in Orlando, Florida, as his first race. He gave himself 4 months to prepare. "I cried the entire way," Coleman confesses about participating in the event. After that first taste of racing, he graduated to races of other distances, including half marathons and full marathons. "I'm fully hooked on the running lifestyle," he says. "And it started with a short run and walk down the block."

Donna Johnson Pittman, 45, a college professor from Clarksville, Tennessee, found her inspiration on the bulletin board of her local YMCA: "I saw a flyer for a local 5K," Pittman recalls. Her initial thought was, "I wonder how far 5K is?" (She soon learned that 5K is 3.1 miles.) It was the middle of June; the 5K was in the middle of October. Deciding that surely she could be ready by then, she walked straight from the bulletin board to an aisle of treadmills and hopped on one. "I cranked up the speed to a running pace and off I went. I only made it a quarter mile. I couldn't breathe. I felt like I was dying. But I became a runner that day. The next day I did it again. And the next day, and for days and days after that. Running changed my life."

ARE YOU A RUNNER?

Do you need to race to call yourself a runner? Not really. In fact, as I look out the window of my Long Beach, Indiana, office onto Lake Shore Drive, which

Do you need to race to call yourself a runner? Not really. serves as a superhighway for runners, walkers, and cyclists, I sometimes think runners who race might even be in the minority, second in numbers to runners who run but never race, not even in local events such as the Old School Run. The number of runners who do not race remains totally unknown to the statisticians at Running USA.

THE RACING SCENE: BEFORE YOU GO

Fearful about showing up at a large road race—or even a small road race? The racing scene is a lot less scary than you might think. Here are some tips that will help you prepare for your first 5K.

■ **Carefully select your first 5K.** In theory, there should be less pressure at a small, local race—that is, unless everybody there knows you. One plus of picking a large race for your first starting-line appearance is anonymity. No one will care how fast (or slow) you run except you.

■ **Learn all about the race.** Find the race Web site. All but the smallest 5K races have Web sites telling all you need to know about the event: Time. Place. Course map. Cost. Read everything you find online. *Everything!* You need to discover all the details about the race: starting time, directions on how to get there, course map, and the like. The more you know, the more comfortable you'll feel at your first 5K.

■ **Enter early.** The most popular races often limit the number accepted into the field. Wait too long and you may find the race closed. More important, filing your entry exhibits a commitment and provides you with the goal you need, plus the entry fee often is less.

■ **Pick a side event.** Many high-profile running events at longer distances (half and full marathons) include secondary "fitness runs" with no times or prizes, thus less pressure to perform. You can

Nevertheless, running a fast time in a 5K and comparing it a few months or even years later to a time in a previously run 5K can be an important motivational tool. It can get you started. It can get you off the couch. It can get you out the door and down the street. It can signal a new beginning, a new you, the birth of a person you never knew existed. The lure of the race and the accompanying race T-shirt, not to mention a medal hung around your neck, definitely can motivate you to participate in an activity that is

enjoy all the fun of the main event without feeling like you are in a race (as our friend Mary Ellen discovered).

■ **Do some scouting.** Attend a major race first as a spectator. Observe with an unbiased mind everything you see, from the start to the finish to the post-race parties. Running races have their rituals. Seeing how smoothly the sport functions will ease your mind.

■ **Plan what to take.** Most runners like to plan what outfit to wear, including shoes, well in advance. Lay your gear out the night before so you don't forget anything, especially your race number. In fact, pin it to your singlet the night before, then try on that singlet to make sure the number fits comfortably. Yes, prerace paranoia is common among runners, novice and experienced alike. Plan for all kinds of weather. Most runners come dressed to run, but you will want to take some extra clothes for postrace activities.

■ **Enjoy the expo.** This is a day-before-the-race extravaganza where runners pick up their bibs (running numbers) and race T-shirts. Expos are fun meeting grounds for runners young and old, novice and expert. As you will quickly learn, the excitement begins long before runners arrive at the starting line.

■ **Don't forget to train.** Most of my shorter-distance training programs last 8 weeks. That guarantees that you will show up at the starting line ready to run.

both fun and good for your health. If you didn't think so, you probably would not have selected a book that is titled Run Fast.

Sooner or later, most runners want to test their newfound fitness in a race, typically a 5K or a 10K. A decade or so ago, it became trendy for new runners to set their sights firmly on the marathon: 26.2 miles. Even the 13.1 miles of the half marathon was not enough to prove their worth. Based on comments by people who follow me on Facebook, I suspect that most runners attempt a shorter distance race before they jump into the marathon. If they follow one of my 18-week training programs, they will encounter my suggestion that they run a half marathon in Week 9 or Week 10. I also suggest they test their legs in a 5K race before embarking on a demanding 18-week program in preparation for a marathon.

Not much serious training is required to finish a 5K: perhaps three or four workouts a week over a period of several weeks. (See the Basic Beginning training programs that start on page 20.) Simply logging an average of a dozen miles a week will do the trick. That does not mean you will finish a 5K near the front, but you will finish.

Should you at least be able to run the full distance of the race chosen (5K or beyond) in a workout to prove that you can do it on race day? You can, but it's not absolutely mandatory. Most marathoners, for example, run no farther than 20 miles in a climactic "long run" session before attempting the entire distance of 26 miles on race day.

If you can cover 2 or more miles in practice two or three times a week over a period of a half dozen or more weeks, without coming totally unglued, the spirit of the race day moment should carry you across the finish line of a 5K—as long as you start slowly and keep a steady pace. (Reaching a 10K finish line requires slightly more training mileage.)

Once you've finished your first race, however, you will most likely find that a new goal beckons. You will realize that it is no longer enough for you to merely cover the distance; you will want to cover it progressively faster. You will enter the world of performance, complete with training logs, lightweight racing shoes, fancy electronic devices, and inside advice from experts like me in an effort to shave seconds and even minutes from your PR.

SETTING PRS

The term PR is part of the running jargon; it means Personal Record. (Some runners use PB, or Personal Best.) Few of us will ever set a world or national record, but anybody can establish a PR. Any time you record a time over any distance (even odd distances in training) it becomes your PR. Every time you run that course or that same distance, you will have an opportunity to improve upon that PR. You can establish PRs for different milestones, like a change in the calendar year or when you move from one age group (35 to 39) to another (40 to 44). Going after PRs can be fun and, perhaps more important, they can be motivational.

There is a downside to constantly chasing PRs, however. As you become more involved in improving your performances, setting new PRs may not always be easy—or advisable. To improve, runners gradually increase their training mileage, the quality of their training sessions, or both. Eventually, however, they risk losing that initial feeling of joy and find that their performances have inexplicably leveled off. Often, aging is the most important factor when it comes to declining performances, but motivation also can fade. This performance plateau can sometimes confront novice runners with this perplexing, diabolical question: are they training too little, or too much?

Jack Daniels, PhD, an exercise physiologist and coach at the State University of New York at Cortland, writes, "Almost anyone can stay happy and injury-free simply by jogging a couple of miles a day. Fine. But these same runners would be even happier if they could run faster. That's simply human nature. We want to get better, and that brings us face to face with the quintessential training question: How can you train hard enough to improve, but not so hard that you get burned out and/or injured?"

The rest of this book will provide an answer to the question just posed by Dr. Daniels. Let's pause and consider your first PR. To establish that benchmark time, you will need to run some distance—any distance—but let's begin with the 5K.

RUN YOUR FIRST 5K

How much do you need to train to be able to run your first 5K race? Most individuals who possess a reasonably high level of fitness (because they bicycle or swim or participate in other sports that involve cardiovascular development) could probably go out and run 3.1 miles on very little training. They might be sore for a few days after the race, but they still could finish.

But if you've made the decision to run a 5K race, you might as well do it

THE RACING SCENE: YOUR BIG DAY

You may feel out of place the first time you appear at a 5K race. This is natural. It happens whenever we do something new and don't understand the so-called rules. Rest assured that every other runner you see has had a "first race" experience. They didn't know what to expect the first time they walked onto a street full of runners. Here are a few tips to help make your first 5K enjoyable.

■ **Arrive early.** You do not want to get stuck in traffic. All the close parking spaces will be gone. Make sure you have time for prerace necessities, which include porta-potty visits (smelly but necessary). Arriving early allows time to absorb the prerace excitement.

■ **Pin your number on the front.** In track meets, athletes often wear numbers on their backs; in road races, they wear numbers on the front. A number pinned to the back will brand you as an R-O-O-K-I-E. You don't want that to happen, do you? Pack a couple of extra safety pins to make sure you can secure your number at all four corners.

■ **Be visible.** If friends plan to accompany you, will they be able to spot you during the race and find you after the race? Wearing a bright race uniform may help. Checking the race map may allow you and your friends to determine good spectator spots and meet-later points. Advertise yourself on Facebook to be sure that everyone knows your plans.

■ **Follow the leader.** In those last few minutes before the start, nobody is going to be watching you. You watch them. When right. The 5K Novice training schedule that follows will help you get race ready. It is only a slight increase from the Basic Beginning schedules in the previous chapter and features a running option for Mondays and a few more miles on Tuesdays and Thursdays. The most important difference is what appears on the seventh day of Week 8: a 5K race. You would be surprised how much difference having a specific goal makes when it comes to focusing your training. When following a goalless program, skipping a workout here or there seems like no big deal. When following a goal-oriented training

everybody starts moving toward the starting line, that's your cue too. It is okay to behave like a lemming, following everybody without shame.

■ **Start in back.** Don't make the mistake of starting near the front, otherwise you'll spend the first mile watching everybody run past you. Start toward the back. You may lose some time crossing the starting line, particularly in big races, but time isn't important to you in your first race—or shouldn't be. With most races timed electronically these days, the clock will start for you only after you cross the starting line, and then stop when you cross the finish line.

■ **Pace yourself.** One reason for starting in back is to avoid running the first mile too fast, either because of enthusiasm or because faster runners pull you along. Once you cross the starting line, settle into your normal training pace—or run even slower. You'll enjoy your first race more if you run comfortably and see what's happening.

■ **Savor the moment.** Every beginner's first race is a special moment. You will experience other running highs as you continue in the sport, but do your best to enjoy your first 5K as much as you can.

With these tips in mind, you should be able to approach your first starting line comfortably. After the start, it's all up to you.

The 5K Novice

WEEK	MON	TUE	WED	THU	FRI	SAT	SUN
1	Rest or run/walk	1.5 mile run	Rest or run/walk	1.5 mile run	Rest	1.5 mile run	30 min walk
2	Rest or run/walk	1.75 mile run	Rest or run/walk	1.5 mile run	Rest	1.75 mile run	35 min walk
3	Rest or run/walk	2 mile run	Rest or run/walk	1.5 mile run	Rest	2.0 mile run	40 min walk
4	Rest or run/walk	2.25 mile run	Rest or run/walk	1.5 mile run	Rest	2.25 mile run	45 min walk
5	Rest or run/walk	2.5 mile run	Rest or run/walk	2.0 mile run	Rest	2.5 mile run	50 min walk
6	Rest or run/walk	2.75 mile run	Rest or run/walk	2.0 mile run	Rest	2.75 mile run	55 min walk
7	Rest or run/walk	3 mile run	Rest or run/walk	2.0 mile run	Rest	3.0 mile run	30 min walk
8	Rest or run/walk	3 mile run	Rest or run/walk	2.0 mile run	Rest	Rest	5K race

program, missing a workout is a big deal. Miss too many workouts, and you compromise the end result: your ability to run fast.

The 5K Novice training program is designed to get you to both the starting line and the finish line of a 5K race. Following this program for the prescribed 8 weeks will teach you to run. Once you have mastered that, I will teach you to run fast.

CHAPTER FIVE

LEVELS OF STRESS: 5K INTERMEDIATE

You need to learn to run slow and build your base before you run fast

O ne of the more successful American track distance runners in recent years has been Amy Begley, a 2008 Olympian. In 2009, Begley finished sixth at the IAAF World Championships, setting a personal record for 10,000 meters of 31:13.78. During her peak years, Begley trained under the supervision of Alberto Salazar, coach of the Nike Oregon Project.

In 2014, the 21,000-member Atlanta Track Club appointed Begley as its first full-time coach. (Her husband, Andrew, also serves as a coach for the club.) As a teenager, Begley ran for East Noble High School in Kendallville, Indiana, a small town of about 10,000 people in the northeast corner of the state. Because I live in Indiana, my connection to Begley goes way back. I remember Begley winning four Indiana state championships: once in cross-country and three times in track as a 3200-meter runner.

Despite competing in distances from 2 to 6 miles, Begley routinely would go for long runs under Salazar's supervision of distances that ranged between 12 and 22 miles, often running significantly slower than her race pace on the track. She now uses the same approach while training runners at the Atlanta Track Club, explaining: "We rotate easy long runs (60 to 75 seconds slower than 10K race pace) with shorter and faster runs (around 30 to 45 seconds slower than 10K pace). Typically, these faster runs are progressive: starting off with an easy jog and easing into the planned pace." She adds, "Only during marathon training, the progressive runs might dip down to race pace. I did workouts with Alberto like this."

Run slower than race pace? This would seem to contradict the mantra for this book and the comment by world champion Lynn Jennings that if you want to run fast, you have to run fast. I'm not going to sell out Jennings. You do have to run fast, provided that your fast training is done at the right time of the year. But another adage says that you can't run fast unless you first train far. And before you run far, you have to develop a level of conditioning and fitness that allows you to run 4 or 5 or 6 or 7 miles or more without exhausting yourself.

AEROBIC BASE

Runners new and experienced need a base of long-distance training. You need a certain number of miles on your legs. I'm not talking about new runners who generally max out in their training programs with "long" runs of 2 to 3 miles. I'm talking about more experienced runners who want to run faster. In my training programs, they would probably be classified as "intermediate" runners.

For intermediate runners, they (or you) need to include runs that go well beyond the 5K or even 10K race distances in their workout week. My training programs for the 5K max out at 7 miles for intermediate runners and 9 miles (or 90 minutes at a 10:00 pace) for advanced runners. When training for a certain number of minutes rather than miles, faster runners may go a mile or two more. My 10K programs max out at 8 miles for intermediate runners and 10 miles for advanced runners.

You need to get in shape before you're ready to compete.

Here's an important point: You need to get in shape before you're ready to compete. That's basic to all sports. In baseball terms, you need to reach first base before you can cross home plate. Melvin H. Williams, PhD, an exercise physiologist at Old Dominion University in Norfolk, Virginia, and a top-ranked masters runner, believes that base training is vital to success in running at any distance.

"Over a long period of time, even small numbers of miles add up to large numbers," says Dr. Williams. "I was never a distance runner in high school, but I always ran to get in shape for other sports. I continued running in the military, and after discharge ran mainly to stay in shape. All that background running helped to lay a groundwork of base training that I took advantage of immediately when I got serious about being a runner."

For all runners, success depends on the development of a strong aerobic base. You need to gradually improve your body's ability to move oxygen from your lungs to your legs. Endurance is the foundation of your running performance. That's true even for sprinters running 100 and 200 meters.

The fastest sprinters are not always those fastest out of the blocks, but rather those who slow down the least in the later stages of the race. "Endurance training must come first," insists Bill Dellinger, former track coach at the University of Oregon in Eugene and a bronze medal winner in the 1964 Olympic Games. "Speed is merely a supplement to strength."

If you are a beginning runner, that means gradually increasing the distance of your daily runs from 1 to 2 to 3 miles or more and eventually including a weekend long run of a somewhat longer distance, such as 4 to 6 miles. Even with such a simple program, great gains can be made in fitness, strength, and speed. You can develop endurance by taking long runs—and for a beginner, even 4 miles can be a long run.

Benji Durden, a 1980 Olympic marathoner and now a coach in Boulder, Colorado, says, "One thing I strongly believe in is the value of a long run. A lot of people, when trying to run fast, overlook the need for strength. There's great value in the weekly long run. If you're pointing for a short race, you still need to run long in training. Just because you're not running more than 2 hours in a race, that doesn't mean that runs that long have no value in your training program."

Russell H. Pate, PhD, director of the human performance laboratory at the University of South Carolina in Columbia and a past president of the

American College of Sports Medicine says, "You need to burn lots of calories to succeed in running, even at modest intensities."

However, Dr. Pate admits that there's a certain risk to that kind of training. "The long run, particularly, can be overdone if done too often or too long. Once a week worked well with me. There are both physiological and psychological benefits to the long run that we can't always measure in the laboratory. Only in the long run do you encounter the muscle glycogen depletion (energy burn) that occurs in competition. There are some adaptions with that form of training that are difficult to get any other way."

He concedes that this theory may be controversial. "Some physiologists might challenge me on that. But when you get into a glycogen-depleted state, you have to make greater use of fat as an energy source. It's probably advantageous to experience what that means in training. Having been there before on a regular basis helps. It also helps from a psychological point of view. You have to tune your mind to focus intently on your running for a long period, whether that period is 30 minutes or 3 hours. That's why long runs are critical to success in any training program, even for distances shorter than the 5K," says Dr. Pate.

HOW LONG IS LONG?

How far should you run? How long is long? Those aren't easy questions to answer, not merely for beginners but also for intermediate and advanced runners. Let's talk about ways you can improve as a runner.

Exercise physiologist Jack Daniels, PhD, states, "To improve your running capabilities, you need to impose a stress that is not an overstress."

Huh? How can a stress not be an overstress? But think about what Dr. Daniels said for a minute. It's a very important point.

It means runners have to be very cautious when it comes to increasing workload. "You want to create a positive reaction to stress, not a negative one," explains Dr. Daniels.

What do I mean by stress? I define stress as anything that gets you out of breath or pushes you out of your comfort zone. Selecting the correct dose of exercise stress is no easy task, either for a runner or for a coach. If you run 20 miles a week and do it for 1 month, what do you do next? Do you shift to 25 miles? To 30? Should you set your sights on 40 weekly miles? Guess wrong and you might get injured—or experience training burnout, which will similarly detract from your performances.

According to Dr. Daniels, "When you go from zero running to 20 miles a week, you'll achieve enormous gains in fitness and your ability to perform. Doubling your mileage from 20 miles to 40 will result in nowhere near that much improvement. It's a case of diminishing returns. The more and more you do, the tougher it is to improve—and at some point, the curve tips downward. So be cautious in increasing workload."

The same applies to intensity. If you run the same number of miles but at a faster pace, you're also increasing your stress load. Whether mileage or intensity, Dr. Daniels advises to limit any increases in stress to every third or fourth week. "Allow yourself time to adjust to a certain amount of stress before imposing another," he suggests.

One way to determine your mileage progression is to decide how many miles you want to be running at peak performance. (When I design training programs, such as those you see in this book, this is where I invariably begin and I then work backward.) If you want to run 40 miles and you're currently running 20 miles, you can achieve that mileage by following Dr. Daniels's lead and add 5 miles to your training program every 4th week. My recipe might call for adding 1 mile every week, but the effect is about the same. You can go from 20 miles to 25 to 30 to 35 to an ultimate 40 weekly miles and theoretically do it in 16 weeks (or 4 months). If you have 6 to 8 months, you can pick a gentler progression and decrease your risk of injury.

"Determining levels of stress," says Dr. Daniels, "is one of the most difficult tasks for any coach or athlete."

Running long and slow is a good way to develop your endurance base, but in terms of developing speed, a danger exists if you train only with long runs. You risk developing the gait and the rhythm of the long-distance runner who becomes efficient at running slowly for a long period of time. That is, your stride may change and you could potentially lose speed.

As a result, you will no longer be able to run fast at shorter distances in an efficient way.

"The major disadvantage of concentrating on volume in training is that long, slow distance training is considerably slower than racing pace," states David L. Costill, PhD. "Such training fails to develop the neurological patterns of muscle fiber recruitment that will be needed during races that require a faster pace. Because the selective use of muscle fibers differs according to running speed, runners who train only at speeds slower than race pace will not train all of the muscle fibers that they need for competition." The best method for developing speed, therefore, is to first develop and maintain a slow base, then move on to faster training.

> *"Determining levels of stress is one of the most difficult tasks for any coach or athlete."*

THE HEART OF THE MATTER

To run fast, you must have a cardiovascular system that is capable of delivering oxygen efficiently. Within certain limits, the more oxygen your muscles receive, the faster you can run. Scientists don't entirely understand the reasons why, but an efficient oxygen delivery system—aerobic base—is best developed by training within 70 to 85 percent of your maximum heart rate (MHR).

When a runner moves beyond 85 percent of his MHR, he or she crosses the anaerobic threshold, or lactate threshold, and experiences different physiological effects. By training anaerobically (intense exercise where oxygen levels are insufficient and your body seeks energy from your muscles), you can develop your ability to readily release energy from your muscles. But you must possess a solid aerobic base first. Without this base, you won't be able to deliver oxygen to your muscles, and your performances will diminish.

Dr. Costill describes anaerobic threshold as the point during exercise when the metabolism supposedly switches from an aerobic to an anaerobic state, when the body's demand for oxygen exceeds its ability to produce it. "Since lactic acid tends to be produced by the muscles when they are unable

AEROBIC VERSUS ANAEROBIC

The best method for developing speed is to begin with a slow aerobic base (exercise where a sufficient level of oxygen intake provides energy), then move to the fast anaerobic training (intense exercise where oxygen levels are insufficient and your body seeks energy from your muscles). A slow run that you can sustain over a period of time is an aerobic activity, whereas an anaerobic activity consists of short bursts of high intensity exercise, such as sprinting.

to acquire sufficient oxygen to produce energy aerobically, its accumulation in the blood is considered to be a good indicator of the pace that the runner can tolerate during long runs," says Dr. Costill.

Robert H. Vaughan, PhD, who coached world-class distance runner and Olympian Francie Larrieu Smith, described this in his doctoral dissertation at the University of North Texas in Denton. Dr. Vaughan noticed that some of the runners he coached were more capable than others of maintaining their competitive ability over a longer period of time. One was Larrieu Smith, who set personal records at the 1988 Olympic Trials in July, then ran faster 2 months later at the Olympic Games in Seoul, Korea, where she placed fifth in the 10,000 meters. (Larrieu Smith went on to make five Olympic teams and carry the US flag into the stadium at the 1992 Olympic Games in Barcelona, Spain.)

Looking back on Larrieu Smith's training, Dr. Vaughan realized that one key to her consistency was that she had maintained her aerobic base by running regular 20-mile workouts, even while preparing for a race one-third that distance. Larrieu Smith was training for seemingly selfish reasons, though. Not only was she primed for the Olympics, she also was looking 5 weeks beyond the Games to running in the Columbus Marathon. Theoretically, training for this marathon could have had a negative effect on Larrieu Smith's Olympic performance; in actuality, it was one of the reasons she ran so well in Seoul.

Larrieu Smith's long runs maintained her aerobic base and, in effect, kept her oxygen delivery system open. With this sound base, she was better able to benefit from the anaerobic (speed) training she also was doing. Other runners coached by Dr. Vaughan did primarily anaerobic training and found that without as sound an aerobic base, they could not maintain their peak conditioning that long into the season. They could run fast, but they could not continue to run fast for weeks and months into a long season.

ADDING MORE DISTANCE

Assuming that you followed the 5K Novice training schedule (page 34) and competed in your first race at that distance, how do you improve? The next step upward is the 5K Intermediate plan. This training will take you to the next level and, with a few more miles in the mix, help you build the aerobic base that will allow you to train anaerobically down the road, so to speak. The 5K Intermediate plan gently increases your distance but it also includes

EVEN PACE

Russian coach A. Yakimov explains how running slow can help you run fast—as long as you do it at an even pace: "At first, it was thought that long, continuous running helped perfect only the aerobic processes, but specialists have since come to the conclusion that it also helps develop the anaerobic potentials of the runner."

Yakimov suggests that coaches and runners be very careful in selecting both the speed and duration of the run. Yakimov wrote in *Track Technique*, "The problem is that the athlete must be able to distribute his effort in order to run the whole way at an even pace. If the pace drops off at the end, the problem has not been solved."

In other words, a workout that starts fast and finishes slow (because of fatigue) may fail to train the muscles properly, either in developing base or in developing speed. Learn to monitor your pace carefully.

some speedwork. "The secret to success," suggests Larry Mengelkoch, PhD, an exercise scientist at the University of St. Augustine for Health Services in Florida, "is to be consistent in your training and not attempt sudden jumps. With moderate intensity, you'll see gradual improvements and can avoid injury."

As we move from the 5K: Novice to the 5K: Intermediate, let me explain some common running terms (many of them shown in the training plan that follows) so you'll know the difference, for instance, between "3 mile run" and "3 mile fast."

Run. When the schedule says "run," it is a suggestion for you to run at an easy pace. How fast is easy? I can't answer that question. You need to define your own comfort level. Don't worry about how fast you run; just cover the distance suggested—or approximately the distance. Ideally, you should be able to run at a pace that allows you to converse with a training partner without getting too much out of breath.

Fast. For several of the Saturday runs, I suggest that you run "fast." How fast is "fast"? Again, that depends on your comfort level. Go somewhat faster than you would on a "run" day. If you are doing this workout right, it should be difficult to converse with your training partner. It's okay now to get out of breath.

Long Runs. Once a week, go for a long run. Not as long as if you were training for a marathon, but longer than your goal race (5K) distance. Run 5 to 7 miles at a comfortable pace, not worrying about pace per mile. Stay in your comfort zone. Don't be afraid to stop to walk or stop to drink. This should be an enjoyable workout, not one during which you punish yourself.

Interval Training. To improve speed, you sometimes need to train at a pace faster than your race pace for the 5K, about the pace you would run in a 1500 meter or mile race. Run 400 meters hard, then recover by jogging and/or walking 400 meters. Before starting this workout, warm up by jogging a mile or two, stretching, and doing a few sprints of 100 meters. Cool down afterward with a short jog.

Tempo Runs. This is a continuous run with an easy beginning, a buildup in the middle to near your 5K race pace, and then an easing back with a cruise to the finish. A typical tempo run would begin with 5 to 10 minutes easy running (warm-up), continue with 10 to 15 minutes faster running, and finish with 5 to 10 minutes easy running (cooldown). Listen to your body to determine your pace. Tempo runs are very useful for developing anaerobic threshold, which is essential for fast 5K racing.

Rest. You can't train hard unless you are well rested. The 5K: Intermediate training schedule includes two designated days for rest: Mondays and Fridays. The easy 3-mile runs scheduled for Tuesdays and Thursdays are designed to complement the harder workout on Wednesdays and over the weekend. The final week before the 5K is a light week. Taper your training so that you can be ready for a peak performance on the weekend.

Stretch and Strengthen. An important addendum to any training program is stretching. Don't overlook it—particularly on days when you plan to run fast. Strength training is important too: do pushups and pullups, use free weights, or work out with various machines at the gym. Runners generally benefit if they combine light weights with a high number of repetitions, rather than pumping very heavy iron. Tuesdays and Thursdays would be good days to combine strength training with your easy run, although you can schedule these workouts on any day that is convenient for your personal schedule.

Racing. Some racing is useful in helping you to peak. Consider doing some other races at 5K to 10K distances to test your fitness. The 5K Intermediate training schedule includes a test 5K race halfway through the program. You could race more frequently (once every 2 weeks), but too much racing is never a good idea.

The 5K Intermediate

WEEK	MON	TUE	WED	THU	FRI	SAT	SUN
1	Rest	3 mile run	5 × 400	3 mile run	Rest	3 mile run	5 mile run
2	Rest	3 mile run	30 min tempo	3 mile run	Rest	3 mile fast	5 mile run
3	Rest	3 mile run	6 × 400	3 mile run	Rest	4 mile run	6 mile run
4	Rest	3 mile run	35 min tempo	3 mile run	Rest	Rest	5K test
5	Rest	3 mile run	7 × 400	3 mile run	Rest	4 mile fast	6 mile run
6	Rest	3 mile run	40 min tempo	3 mile run	Rest	5 mile run	7 mile run
7	Rest	3 mile run	8 × 400	3 mile run	Rest	5 mile fast	7 mile run
8	Rest	3 mile run	30 min tempo	2 mile run	Rest	Rest	5K race

This training schedule is only a guide. If you want to do long runs on Saturday rather than Sunday, simply flip-flop the days. If you have an important appointment on a day when you have a hard workout planned, do a similar switch with a rest day. Feel free to make minor modifications to suit your work and family schedule. It's less important what you do in any one workout than what you do over the full 8 weeks leading up to your 5K.

CHAPTER SIX

RUN SLOW
Speed training without speedwork

Were I a carnival barker, I might stand on a box with a copy of this book in my hand and chant: "I am going to give you a secret workout guaranteed to take minutes off your times—at any distance!" That same pitch might easily work on the cover of *Runner's World* magazine: "Secret Speed: Easy Route to a PR!" Getting closer to revealing this secret, I could offer a 139-character tweet: "Speedwork is only one training method if you want to run fast. You can get to the finish line of your next 5K faster if you also run slow."

Really, Hal? Yes, you have the right to question the veracity of my carnival barker pitch. But let me explain, using the scientific advisement of one of the world's all-time great middle-distance runners, New Zealand's Peter Snell, PhD, who is also an associate professor of internal medicine at the University of Texas.

While training for the 1960 Olympic Games, Dr. Snell ran with veteran Murray Halberg on an extremely hilly 22-mile loop in Owairaka on the outskirts of Auckland, New Zealand. At that time, Dr. Snell was an up-and-coming 800-meter runner; Halberg was a veteran miler, moving up to the 5000 meters. Considering their specialty distances, the Owairaka loop (still renowned among distance buffs) seemed like an excessive amount of miles. The pace, much slower than his racing pace, both fatigued and frustrated Dr. Snell.

"I'm going to stop at 15 miles," he finally told Halberg.

Halberg warned the younger runner not to quit. "If you stop now, you'll completely waste the value of this workout. You have to run 15 miles before reaping the benefits that come in the last 7."

Dr. Snell was not entirely convinced, but he persevered through that workout and other long, slow training runs prescribed by his coach, Arthur Lydiard. At the 1960 Olympics that summer in Rome, the unheralded Kiwi astonished everybody by winning the 800 meters in a record 1:46.3. Halberg, his training partner, won the 5000 meters. Four years later, Dr. Snell won both the 800 and 1500 meters at the 1964 Olympic Games in Tokyo. In between, he set world records of 3:54.4 for the mile and of 1:44.3 for the 800 that surprised him even more than it did track fans.

"It was a total shock because I had done almost no fast training leading up to that race," Dr. Snell later would tell me. "I spent most of the winter running slow workouts. I even ran a marathon in about 2:30 as part of my practice! After the marathon, I went to the track, added some speed training, and boom: world record. I couldn't believe at the time that you could learn to run fast by running slow."

"If you stop now, you'll completely waste the value of this workout."

After Dr. Snell retired from competition, he moved to the United States to study for a degree in exercise physiology at Washington State University under Phil Gollnick, PhD. Dr. Snell came to recognize the scientific principles that permitted him to use slow running to train his predominantly fast-twitch muscles.

In 1974, Dr. Gollnick collaborated on a study with Bengt Saltin, PhD, one of Sweden's top exercise physiologists. Dr. Gollnick and Dr. Saltin studied a group of cyclists in their laboratories. They took muscle biopsies of the cyclists as they exercised and discovered that after 60 or 90 minutes, most of the glycogen stored in the cyclists' slow-twitch muscles had become depleted. (Glycogen is the form of glucose, or sugar, stored in the muscles that serves as fuel.)

Slow-twitch muscles are used most often in aerobic endurance activities;

A QUICK SCIENCE LESSON

Through the use of muscle biopsies (slicing out a miniscule piece of muscle and examining it under a microscope), exercise scientists have been able to divide muscles into two distinct types: fast twitch and slow twitch. Fast-twitch muscles fire quickly but also tire quickly; slow-twitch muscles react more slowly but do not fatigue as easily. Not too surprisingly, most sprinters have a preponderance of fast-twitch muscles, while distance runners most often have more slow-twitch muscles.

It's one of the reasons why Jamaica's Usain Bolt was able to dominate sprinting at the world level for nearly a decade, not merely setting world records at 100 and 200 meters, but *crushing* the previous world records. Could Bolt translate that speed from the shortest Olympic distances to the longest Olympic distance, the marathon? No. Conversely, top marathoners such as Wilson Kipsang and Meb Keflezighi who dominate that distance would be unable to challenge Bolt in his specialty.

Most of us fit somewhere in the middle when it comes to fast twitch versus slow twitch. Other factors notwithstanding, some people are born to be better 5K runners; others, to be better marathoners. Training can affect some changes, and indeed one subcategory of fast-twitch muscles can be trained more for endurance than another category.

How well fast-twitch and slow-twitch muscles perform depends partly on how much fuel is available during exercise. Both muscle types burn fuel to function well. Glycogen is the most efficient form of fuel for energy. Glycogen is a substance similar to sugar that is most easily stored in the muscles when you consume carbohydrates. Fats and proteins also can be converted into energy, though less efficiently. When glycogen becomes depleted, performance results diminish, even in short-distance races such as the 5K. Glycogen depletion is one reason why some marathoners "hit the wall" 20 miles into their 26-mile races.

fast-twitch muscles are used more for anaerobic speed activities. (See the sidebar, "A Quick Science Lesson.") With glycogen depleted from the slow-twitch muscles, the cyclists' bodies began to recruit the fast-twitch muscles for their supplies of additional glycogen. As a result, Dr. Gollnick and Dr. Saltin discovered, the body "trained" these fast-twitch muscles.

"When I reviewed the results of the Gollnick and Saltin study," says Dr. Snell, "I finally realized what Murray meant when he said the 'benefits' of our 22-mile run at Owairaka didn't begin until we had gone 15 miles. Murray was no exercise scientist—and neither was our coach Lydiard—but both realized instinctively that by pushing into that netherworld of glycogen depletion, you could actually improve your speed as well as your endurance."

BANISHING SPEEDWORK

Although the Gollnick and Saltin study was completed many decades ago, competitive athletes from high school cross-country runners to world-class track stars have used various forms of long, slow distance (LSD) running to prepare for their competitive seasons. But the adult runners who might most benefit from long, slow running have not always understood how jogging along at a gentle pace might help them run faster and set PRs at popular distances such as the 5K or 10K.

When counseling marathon runners online, I often suggest that they do their long runs at a tempo that is 30 to 90 seconds (or more) slower than their goal marathon pace. In fact, I emphasize the "or more," saying that I don't care how slow they do their long runs. This perplexes some runners who wonder how they can be expected to maintain a certain pace in the marathon itself if they don't run that pace in practice. (The answer is by doing separate "pace runs," but that's another subject.) I usually don't need to spend much time defending my statement, because other runners post comments about their own experiences, comments that can be summarized by the simple statement, "It works!"

Certainly, articles in *Runner's World* magazine and various books (including previous editions of this one) have popularized the idea that if you want to maximize your ability at shorter distances, you need to do speedwork: interval training on the track, hill repeats, fartlek, and demanding tempo runs near race pace. (Is that not the mantra of this book: If you want to run fast, you have to run fast?)

Those training methods still work, but they don't work equally for all runners. Not everybody is capable of pounding out a series of fast quarter-miles or hill repeats without getting injured. Many individuals are unfortunately intimidated by the thought of sharing a track with elite athletes. I will venture to say that many of readers of this book will feel relieved at Dr. Snell's message that slow running can help improve their speed.

But just any slow running won't work, suggests Dr. Snell, who reported his theories at a meeting of the American College of Sports Medicine. It must be slow running carried on for a period of 60 to 90 minutes, at which point glycogen becomes depleted from the slow-twitch muscles. It is this slow-twitch depletion that allows the fast-twitch muscles to undergo a similar depletion. It is at this point that the fast-twitch muscles are trained. This process can be enhanced, says Dr. Snell, if the runner then speeds up his pace. (You should still eat normally before long runs. High carb remains the rule.)

During a visit to New Zealand some years ago, I was driven over the famed Owairaka course by the late John Davies, who placed third in the 1964 Olympic 1500 meters behind Dr. Snell. I was able to see firsthand how athletes trained under the direction of Lydiard. Over the first third of the 22-mile distance, they faced a series of climbs culminating in one final, steep ascent to loop through a forest area overlooking the city of Auckland.

This middle third of the run was relatively flat. The final third involved downhill running, since what goes up in a long run eventually must come down, and vice versa. This encouraged Lydiard's runners to increase their pace toward the end of their runs. It was at this point during his workout with Halberg that a younger Dr. Snell had considered stopping.

When Dr. Snell, Halberg, Davies, and Lydiard's other runners trained on the Owairaka course decades ago, it was mostly farmland. By the time Davies showed me the course, farmland had become urban sprawl, an endless stretch of gas stations, housing developments, and shopping centers leading up to the forest. Fewer runners train on the Owairaka course today, and, whether coincidentally or not, New Zealand less often wins medals at

(continued on page 54)

JUNK MILES

They are disparagingly called junk miles—those slow, extra miles done on our easy days or in second workouts, sometimes to inflate training mileage—to be able to say we ran 25 miles last week rather than merely 15, or 50 rather than 45. I certainly plead guilty. During my peak years, I ran twice daily, often dragging myself through extra workouts so I could hit 100 miles a week, an important psychological barrier—or so I thought.

But did those junk miles do me any good? Would increasing your weekly mileage from 20 to 30 to 40 or more make you a better runner or will doing so simply increase your risk of injury? Are junk miles like junk food: burning empty calories with little training effect?

Research shows that junk miles can provide meaningful benefits. For example, one study at the University of Wisconsin–La Crosse by Carl Foster, PhD, showed that athletes' performance improved when they incorporated recovery days that featured so-called junk miles. "You need true recovery days in order to allow the real training to work," says Dr. Foster.

Another study, conducted at the University of Georgia by Michael J. Breus and Patrick O'Connor, PhD, demonstrated that exercising even at 40 percent of maximal capacity significantly lowered anxiety levels, and thus could help prevent staleness. "These results are good news for those who want to get benefits from exercise, but who don't enjoy working out at a high intensity," summarizes Breus.

It's also good news for those of us who enjoy running slow and don't want to feel guilty about not "going all-out" every time we lace up our training shoes. Even so-called junk miles benefit runners in many ways.

■ **Strength.** Running farther increases strength, which also increases speed. "It's the principle of multiple repetitions of a light weight," suggests coach Roy Benson of Amelia Island, Florida. "Every step you run does count."

- **Calorie burn.** Junk miles burn calories as efficiently as fast miles; it just takes longer to burn them. Regardless of pace, each mile you run burns approximately 100 calories for someone weighing 150 pounds.

- **Economy.** Extra miles can make you a more efficient runner. "A low, shuffling stride is faster than a high, bounding stride," says Benson. Run longer miles and you'll improve running economy.

- **Relaxation.** For someone who enjoys running, taking a day off is not an easy training option. "Junk miles on recovery days help prevent runners from becoming depressed and stale," says Dr. O'Connor.

How do you fit junk miles into your training? On days between hard workouts, make sure your pace is slow enough to promote recovery. The same goes for long runs on weekends. Not every workout has to be conducted flat-out fast. Still another approach is to occasionally substitute easy running for cross-training.

The downside to junk miles, however, is that running long and slow can tighten as well as strengthen your muscles. "You need to do more stretching to stay loose," warns Benson. Thus, when adding junk miles to your routine, be sure to do your stretching exercises after each workout.

Also, adding miles to your training should be done on a gradual basis. One rule is to never increase your mileage by more than 10 percent a week—and even that percentage may be too much when your mileage starts soaring past 30 or 40 miles a week. While increasing mileage, occasionally schedule a "stepback" week that features lowered mileage before pushing upward again.

Don't overlook the value of good junk. Don't be shy about including some very slow miles in training, particularly on days between your hard sessions. Cross-training is not always the best option. Can you use junk miles while recovering from an injury? Yes, but rest may make more sense. Your performances can improve if you know when and how to use junk miles.

the Olympic Games. But the training principles that resulted in Dr. Snell's and Halberg's successes remain valid today and can be applied by runners at all levels.

The secret, the Kiwis believed, was to start slow during long runs, but finish fast.

3/1 TRAINING

The contour of the Owairaka course prompted Dr. Snell and his training companions to pick up the pace toward the end. They ran the course every other Sunday, holding back every other week to prevent overtraining. Even if you can't find a course that provides a downhill push at the end, you can adjust your training into a similar slow/fast pattern. The result might be called 3/1 training, an approach favored by Davies. Runners coached by Davies included former world record holders Dick Quax and Anne Audain.

In 3/1 training, you run at a comfortable pace for the first three-fourths of the workout. In the final one-fourth, you gradually accelerate to a pace that is 30 to 90 seconds faster per mile than the pace you had been running. For the typical 20-mile run in preparation for a marathon, this would mean running the first 15 miles at a slow pace, then running faster in the final 5 miles. If running an 8-mile workout, you would pick up the pace for the final 2 miles.

Start slow during long runs, but finish fast.

Of course, you don't have to be a marathoner to benefit from 3/1 training. As Dr. Snell explains—and as the Gollnick and Saltin research demonstrated—you need run only 60 to 90 minutes to deplete the glycogen from your slow-twitch muscles. If you run at a 10-minute pace per mile, you would enter this zone after 6 miles of your 8-mile run. As your body begins to tap your fast-twitch muscles for additional glycogen, you speed up, giving those muscles an extra training boost. In an 8-mile workout, someone running at a 10-minute pace would run the first 60 minutes at that slow pace; the final 20 minutes would be done somewhat faster.

How much faster? It depends on the individual runner and what he or she defines as slow or fast. A runner accustomed to running his longer work-outs at an 8-minute-mile pace might begin by running 8:30 or 9-minute miles, pushing to 7:30 or even 7-minute pace toward the end of the run. For those who use heart monitors to guide them in their training, the first three-fourths of the run might be executed at an easy pace, say 65 to 75 percent of maximum heart rate (MHR), before moving to a medium pace of 75 to 80 percent MHR.

Will adapting 3/1 training allow you to banish speedwork from your bag of workout tricks? If you want to attain peak performance, probably not. But 3/1 training certainly provides a useful addition to any runner's arsenal. The training technique is not revolutionary; Lydiard's runners began using it decades ago. Somewhat revolutionary is the idea that this type of training can be adapted to fit the needs of the majority of runners who do not have their sights on an Olympic gold medal. Regardless of your motives in adapt-ing 3/1 training, it can help you get to your next PR at any race distance.

CHAPTER SEVEN

BREAKTHROUGH: 5K ADVANCED

Sometimes it is possible to make enormous performance jumps

After 25 years as a runner, Frank Walaitis, 50, a teacher from Carpentersville, Illinois, reached the point where continued improvement seemed to have become the impossible dream. His times for the 5K, 10K, half marathon, and full marathon all had flatlined. Walaitis still trained hard, but apparently not hard enough.

Sooner or later, every runner's times flatline. Nobody is immune. When you begin to run, improvement is easy. Step on the escalator. Let it carry you upward to greater levels of glory. For someone possessing zero fitness, each workout brings improvement. Each day dawns with hope and ends with achievement. For many people, the amount of improvement they achieve during the first few weeks and months as a runner is remarkable, spectacular, worthy of praise.

The heart is among the first muscle to react to training; it grows stronger. The strengthened cardiovascular system pushes more and more oxygen-rich blood to the muscles. Simultaneously, the muscles can absorb and burn the oxygen more rapidly, more efficiently, and also push the waste products of combustion out of the system. Fat melts from the body. Less weight equals easier running. Leg muscles also strengthen, allowing the runner to move faster and faster and faster.

Alas, no more for Walaitis, who seemed doomed to accept slower and slower times as age crept upon him.

But wait . . .

For years, Walaitis had done some speedwork. He went to the track now and then, mostly to run mile repeats at a pace near equal to what he might run in marathons. He did so without any particular plan, but eventually began to realize that a program with "some speedwork" performed "now and then" had its limitations.

"My breakthrough came when I became consistent with my quarter-mile repeats," explains Walaitis. "I realized that the only way to run fast was to run faster. Training at marathon pace was not enough. I needed to build from the bottom. I began to run those quarter-mile repeats at 5K race pace. When that pace became comfortable, I pushed myself to the point where I could run those repeats 5 seconds faster."

But a consistent, once-a-week fast running routine was not enough to make a breakthrough. Walaitis added a second speed session each week that featured mile repeats, which over a period of weeks and months became easier and easier. He explains: "I was more fluid in my steps. My recovery between reps was faster. It was like I had found a 'happy place' for my training. Eventually, I was able to run five 1-mile repeats faster than my previous 5K race pace." The extra speedwork allowed Frank to drop 10 minutes from his marathon time, from 3:12 to 3:02. Believe me when I tell you that improvements at that extreme level of fitness, and at that age, do not come easily.

Katherine Barski, 45, an attorney from Palm Beach Gardens, Florida, took a different approach, adding more miles to her training regimen. "For my first marathon, my longest weekly mileage was 30 miles," says Barski. "By the time of my third marathon, I had pushed my weekly mileage up to 50 miles, allowing me to shave 30 minutes off my finishing time." Perhaps even more impressive was that she also cut a half hour off her half marathon time.

To me, the important message that comes from the success of Walaitis and Barski is that if you want to improve, if you want to run faster, you should do something different!

Do something different!

If the focus of your training has been endurance, add speedwork. If the focus of your training has been speedwork, add endurance. Get out of your training rut: *Do something different!* My biggest breakthrough came when I not only increased my dose of speedwork, but also increased the number of miles I ran. I was stationed with the US Army in Germany. In an Olympic year, the Army allowed me to train full time, meaning I could run in the morning, run in the afternoon, and rest in between. Just like the Kenyans. My speedwork diet consisted of multiple repeats at distances between 200 and 1000 meters with fast jogging in between. Over a period of time, I doubled my mileage from 50 miles a week to 100 miles a week. In one year, I sliced nearly a full minute off my time on the track for 5000 meters.

If you want one reason why the East Africans are so fast on both the track and on the roads, it is because the entire focus of their lives—as had been true with me—revolves around running. Few individuals reading this book can afford such a commitment. Nonetheless, they still can improve by making changes in their training focus. Let me say it again: *Do something different!*

That might include other approaches to improvement, as suggested by the following runners I contacted through my Facebook page:

■ **Organization.** Konnie McCollum, Madison, Indiana: "I cut 34 minutes off my marathon time in less than a year by following Hal Higdon's Intermediate 1 Marathon Training plan to the T! I'm running another marathon in two days, and I'm planning on shedding another 10 to 15 minutes or more following the same plan."

■ **Weight loss.** Dominique Gallant, Halifax, Nova Scotia: "Weight loss definitely worked for me. My marathon times went gradually from 5 hours-plus to 4:28 over a period of several years. Then, after a 3-year break, during which time I ran other distances including half marathons, I returned to the marathon, my goal being 4:15 or 4:20. But then I ran a totally unexpected 3:58, followed in another race by a 3:57. This came after losing approximately 20 pounds. I am fairly sure I can attribute a 1-minute improvement for each pound lost."

■ **Smoothies and speedwork.** Sydney Sorkin, Leawood, Kansas: "After having a poor first marathon, I made a decision to improve my nutrition. I always had been bad about eating fruits and veggies. After each workout, I made a fruit smoothie as opposed to previously grabbing whatever food was nearby. I also added a speed workout. Two-and-a-half months after that bad marathon, I got a 5-minute PR in the half marathon and a 20-second PR in the 5K, after more than 2 years of no improvement. 'Smoothies and speedwork' brought the breakthrough for me."

■ **Consistency.** Tommy Snyder, Colfax, Illinois: "I cut over 5 minutes off my 10K time in a year, and I saw similar results at other distances. I feel this breakthrough was the result of three changes: 1. eliminating speedwork and overtraining caused by running too fast; 2. more consistency in training activities; and 3. more miles, possible because running easier eliminated injuries. I would not favor one over the others. All three are directly related."

Blending basic training approaches like these is all part of the balance of being a good runner, of being able finally to run fast, even after years and years of drifting in the doldrums. Yes, ladies and gentlemen, you can achieve a breakthrough. If your training focus has been only on miles run, you may be missing something if you fail to add at least some speed training and appropriate doses of rest, not only between hard workouts but between periods of speed or endurance. And you don't need to go to the track to do interval training (discussed in Chapter 13). Speeding up to race pace in the middle of a workout and then carrying that pace for a mile or even less counts as speedwork.

"A key to running faster is to train faster, wisely; and to think like an athlete."

Listen to Bob Glover, coach for the New York Road Runners. Helen of Troy may have launched a thousand ships with her beauty, but Glover certainly launched a hundred times that number of runners who were bent on personal achievement, specifically success in the New York City Marathon. "A key to running faster is to train faster, wisely; and to think like an athlete. You have to train the body to move faster than you think possible—whether a back-of-the-packer or Olympian. Quicker running improves form and thus efficiency. It makes race pace less daunting."

THE NEXT STEP UPWARD

Let's keep what Glover said in mind as we move upward to the next step in helping you run faster. Having discussed my Novice and Intermediate programs for the 5K in previous chapters, it's time now to consider an Advanced 5K program. Even though you may have no desire to ever run an advanced program with its double dose of speedwork, you would do well to pay attention. The information offered here can help you, no matter your current level or the level you ultimately hope to achieve.

Some of the terms were discussed in earlier chapters, but please allow me to define them again—particularly because advanced runners (given their level of experience) might self-define these terms somewhat differently than novice runners.

Run. The assumption might be that when I say "run," you should go slower than race pace, at a comfortable/conversational level. But sometimes when an advanced runner hits the trails for an easy 3-miler, unless he or she is a slave to his or her GPS watch, that comfortable/conversational pace might actually be faster than race pace. If you can feel the wind in your hair, you may not want to slow down. So don't. Ignore your watch and define your own level of comfort.

Fast. Here is another instructive term where the definition depends on the experiences of the individual runners following my advanced program. Where is the line between fast and slow? Normally, I would suggest race pace. But race pace can be dramatically different depending on whether your goal race is 5K or the marathon. And sometimes in designing workouts, particularly interval training on the track, I might prescribe 1500-meter pace or even 800-meter pace. If you never have run those distances on the track, that may or may not prove helpful to you. I concede that each runner may define "fast" in different ways.

Long runs. A major difference between long runs as presented to advanced runners compared to novice and intermediate runners is that I prescribe time rather than distance. Sunday long runs in the 5K Advanced schedule begin at 60 minutes and peak at 90 minutes. For an experienced runner capable of running miles at a 9:00 mile pace or faster, that would take that runner to 10 miles or beyond. That's okay: If you're training at this level, you should not get hung up on distance.

Interval training. In the 5K Advanced plan, I suggest running 200s and 400s on the track (10 × 200 and 8 × 400 at peak). How fast? Race pace for the 5K would be a good choice. Walk or jog between for some rest, but not total rest. Looking for the best workout for achieving success? Chapter 13 is entirely devoted to interval training. How important do I consider interval training? That I title the chapter "The Magic Workout" is no coincidence.

Tempo runs. This is a gentler form of speedwork than interval training—or it should be if you do it right. Numerous coaches define tempo runs as a workout done at a fast and steady pace, what I might call a fast continuous run (FCR). Because this is my book and these are my programs, I get to define tempo runs here: Begin at an easy jog followed by a gradual acceleration to near race pace in the middle, then finish at an easy jog. Chapter 15 is dedicated to tempo running.

Rest. There's less room for rest at the advanced level. It should come as no surprise that many experienced runners love to run and do not necessarily want to take a day off from running, even on a Friday before a hard weekend of workouts. And to suggest "rest or easy run" on Wednesdays between the two speedwork days, oh my, what is Coach thinking? The reality for runners at this level, however, is that a gentle run even as far as a half-dozen miles might count as rest. We all are different when it comes to our bodies being able to absorb hard training. I find that speed-work works best with easy days before and after, but do what is right for your body.

Racing. I don't include a lot of racing in this schedule: only a 5K test race in Week 4. And you could just as easily run this as a time trial without bothering to pin a number on your chest. If so, then you would train for 8 weeks and cap it with a single 5K race at the end. For some experienced runners, however, even two events may not be enough racing to satisfy them. Would three or four races at various distances diminish their ability to set a PR at the end of Week 8? It just might. Consider the possibility of focusing the entire 8-week period on training, with multiple races coming afterward rather than during.

Here then is my advanced training program leading to a 5K race.

The 5K Advanced

WEEK	MON	TUE	WED	THU	FRI	SAT	SUN
1	3 mile run	5 × 400	Rest or easy run	30 min tempo	Rest	4 mile fast	60 min run
2	3 mile run	8 × 200	Rest or easy run	30 min tempo	Rest	4 mile fast	65 min run
3	3 mile run	6 × 400	Rest or easy run	35 min tempo	Rest	5 mile fast	70 min run
4	3 mile run	9 × 200	Rest or easy run	35 min tempo	Rest or easy run	Rest	5K test
5	3 mile run	7 × 400	Rest or easy run	40 min tempo	Rest	5 mile fast	80 min run
6	3 mile run	10 × 200	Rest or easy run	40 min tempo	Rest	6 mile fast	85 min run
7	3 mile run	8 × 400	Rest or easy run	45 min tempo	Rest	6 mile fast	90 min run
8	2 mile run	6 × 200	30 min tempo	Rest or easy run	Rest	Rest	5K race

CHAPTER EIGHT

SPEED ENDURANCE
Where time meets intensity

Here is a very important point as stated by Russell H. Pate, PhD, chairman of the Department of Exercise Science at the University of South Carolina. Dr. Pate believes that even well-trained runners can improve speed by simply improving endurance. He links the two concepts in a single term: speed endurance.

Dr. Pate—who once ran the marathon in a world-class time of 2 hours, 15 minutes—defines endurance as the ability to continue activity of a designated intensity for a prolonged period. You go far. But speed endurance couples the ability to go far with the ability to go fast. In other words, you attain the ability to go farther faster.

Is your head spinning yet? Let me step out of the way and let you hear from Dr. Pate, who believes that three major physiological factors contribute to speed endurance.

Oxygen uptake. Referring to the maximum volume of oxygen your body can transport and absorb, the term VO_2 max is often used by scientists to describe aerobic power potential—the ability to deliver oxygen to the muscles, particularly for endurance activity. But be careful. Don't confuse this scientists' max with the coaches' max, which more often describes maximum heart rate. (See sidebar "The Two Maxes," below.)

Lactate threshold. Some individuals start to accumulate lactic acid sooner than others. Lactate threshold is the point where lactic acid—produced when the body is working at high effort—begins to accumulate in your bloodstream, which will force you to slow down. "An untrained person may accumulate lactic acid at as low as 30 to 40 percent of their max VO_2," says Dr. Pate. Their

THE TWO MAXES

The term VO_2 max is often used by exercise physiologists as a convenient benchmark to measure human performance, but runners frequently confuse it with another "max" more often used by coaches: maximum heart rate, or MHR.

Your VO_2 max relates to the maximum volume of oxygen transported to your muscles. Usually, scientists obtain the measurement by monitoring athletes while they run on a treadmill or ride an exercise bike, breathing into a device that measures gas volume. This permits researchers to arrive at a figure that defines the amount of oxygen an athlete can consume per kilogram of body weight per minute (ml/kg/min).

Handier is the coaches' max: MHR. Coaches find MHR the best measure of ability, as they are dedicated to training athletes rather than testing them. Maximum heart rate is just what it says. It's the maximum number of times your heart beats under extreme stress, usually measured per minute.

One hundred percent of VO_2 max is the same as 100 percent maximum heart rate, but after that, the two maxes diverge. For instance, to achieve 50 percent of VO_2 max, you actually exercise at 75 percent of your MHR.

It's also possible to achieve levels above 100 percent of VO_2 max, at least for short periods of time. In dealing with MHR, 100 percent is the max. With the exception of this chapter, you'll encounter the term MHR more frequently than VO_2 max in this book because I believe MHR is easier to measure and put to use.

lactate thresholds are very low. "More highly trained endurance athletes, on the other hand, will be able to work at 80 percent or more without accumulating lactic acid." They have developed a high lactate threshold, so they can perform longer and harder at sub-max levels. Dr. Pate notes that VO_2 max sets a cap on the entire system. "I don't think we've ever found an individual who can work for more than a few minutes at 100 percent of max VO_2," he says, "because you start accumulating lactic acid too rapidly."

Efficiency. Efficiency relates to biomechanics and economy of motion. The smoother you are, the less oxygen you consume at a particular running speed. "The lower the rate of oxygen consumption, the lower the amount of metabolic and cardiorespiratory stress and the farther you can run," says Dr. Pate. Efficiency, scientists agree, is most difficult to modify by training. In this case, genetics rules.

"To acquire speed endurance, you need to put these three factors together," Dr. Pate explains. "The optimum would be to have a high VO_2 [max], have a high lactate threshold, and be very economical." A program that develops these three factors produces high-powered performances. Regardless of your level of ability, you can improve by following such a program.

ACQUIRING SPEED ENDURANCE

Some of your endurance capacity is natural. If you possess the ability to endure, it is probably because you have a higher percentage of slow-twitch than fast-twitch muscles. Thus, genes determine our endurance capacity. If you want to be a fast runner, it is often said, carefully select your parents. But to *improve* your base endurance, you need to train. "Anybody, regardless of their muscle composition, can improve endurance with training," says David L. Costill, PhD. To develop speed endurance, you need to use specific types of training. How do you achieve that end? Let's begin by expanding our discussion on developing your base endurance. To do so, I need to use some difficult scientific terms, so please bear with me for a moment.

Improving endurance requires muscle adaptations, claims William Fink, who worked closely with Dr. Costill. The key, says Fink, is producing more mitochondria, a subcellular organelle that makes adenosine triphosphate (ATP), the energy that fuels your muscles. "When someone exercises aerobically," Fink explains, "we see increased activity in a number of specific enzymes involved in the utilization of ATP. The muscle also develops more capillaries, which enhance the delivery of blood and oxygen to the muscle."

According to Stan James, MD, an orthopedic surgeon and cross-country skier from Eugene, Oregon, "There's a certain amount of endurance associated with increased strength, which also comes with endurance training."

Dr. Pate adds, "The muscle develops more connective tissue, a larger cross section. All of this improves endurance."

The key to endurance training, according to Dr. Pate, is to gradually increase your exercise stress. He explains: "In order to induce an adaptation, you have to force the system to do something it is not currently adapted to." Remember what I told you in the previous chapter: If you want to run faster, do something different!

But the amount of stress is specific to each runner. "The trick is to apply a stress sufficient to adapt the system without the undesirable side effects and injuries that come with doing too much. This all needs to be individualized. People vary in how much exercise they can tolerate," says Dr. Pate.

So true. Nevertheless, scientists can now state with some precision how much training is necessary for the average runner to improve endurance, specifically speed endurance. Howard A. Wenger and Gordon J. Bell of the School of Physical Education of the University of Victoria in British Columbia identified three factors necessary to achieve maximal gains in aerobic power, the essential quality of speed endurance. They are intensity, frequency, and duration.

Intensity. According to Wenger and Bell, "The magnitude of change in VO_2 [max] increases as exercise intensity increases from 50 to 100 percent VO_2 [max], and then begins to fall as the intensity exceeds VO_2 [max]."

That statement certainly requires some explanation because of possible confusion between the scientists' max and the coaches' max. To begin to get improvement in your VO_2 max, you must exercise at an intensity equal to at least 50 percent of your VO_2 max. This means you need to train at 75 percent of your maximum heart rate (MHR), a pace that we might call your minimum aerobic pace. (Here's the twist: This means that the better your condition, the harder you need to train to improve your VO_2 max.)

Translation: To improve your endurance, train at 75 percent of your MHR or higher.

Frequency. Wenger and Bell go on to say, "Improvements in VO_2 [max] are greater in both absolute and relative terms up to six sessions per week (for low fitness). In the high-fitness category, however, no improvements are elicited with only two sessions per week, and maximal gains accrue at a frequency of four."

Translation: To improve endurance, train with some intensity (at minimum, this means near race pace) four times a week, approximately every other day.

Duration. Wenger and Bell note some improvements in training sessions of 15 to 30 minutes. They identify the most improvements when exercise exceeds 35 minutes. They write, "This improvement could reflect the greater involvement of fast-twitch motor units as slow-twitch units begin to fatigue."

Beyond 45 minutes, however, improvements decline, most likely because it becomes difficult to maintain intensity (as described previously) for that long a time or to train that hard with the right frequency.

Translation: To improve endurance, the hard portion of your average workout should last 35 to 45 minutes.

To summarize the results of the Wenger and Bell survey: The combination of intensity and frequency that elicits the greatest absolute and relative change is 75 to 90 percent of your MHR four times per week, with an exercise duration of 35 to 45 minutes. The scientists add, however, "It is important to note that lower intensities still produce effective changes and reduce the risks of injury in nonathletic groups."

SMART TRAINING

One of the appeals of an endurance sport such as running, of course, is that you can overcome a lack of natural ability—considered by many the most essential ingredient for athletic success—with dedication and training. Does that statement motivate you? It should. Acquiring speed endurance requires some natural talent, but with the mental focus to train hard—and to train smart—anyone can develop a faster, stronger pace.

You can overcome a lack of natural ability . . . with dedication and training.

Dr. Pate, drawing on both his research as an exercise physiologist and his own experiences as a world-class marathoner, believes that smart training is the key to improving speed endurance. What is smart training? One key factor, he says, is regular pace changes. Here are four different paces that you can use to bring variety to your workouts. For the purposes of this chapter and with Dr. Pate as our instructor, I'm going to divide paces into Pace 1, Pace 2, Pace 3 and Pace 4.

Pace 1: High Intensity

"For decades," says Dr. Pate, "exercise physiologists have studied changes in VO_2 [max], and have learned that you can modify it. I think it's debatable whether or not we know the best way to modify VO_2 [max], but clearly, high-intensity activity is a key. Exercising at intensities that go beyond the individual's current VO_2 [max] is important."

What type of training would this be? Skip back to the start of Chapter 7 and the example of Frank Walaitis, who sliced 10 minutes off his already fast marathon time by increasing the pace of his interval workouts. Walaitis started running his quarter-mile splits at 5K pace instead of marathon pace.

A typical Pace 1 workout would be three 1-mile repeats (3 × mile) at your racing speed, with 5 minutes or more of walking or jogging in between each hard effort. (A "repeat" is any distance run at a set pace, followed by fairly complete rest and more runs at that same distance.) Dr. Pate suggests a speed that is close to your most recent 5K race. A runner capable of a 25:00 5K, for instance, would run his mile repeats at about an 8:00 mile pace.

In designing training schedules, I often use the term "race pace"—which admittedly sometimes confuses beginning runners. They often post questions online like: "What do you mean by race pace?" The answer is fairly simple. Race pace is the pace you plan to run in the race for which you're training. If you're training to run the 5K in 25:00, race pace would be 8:00 per mile for that 3.1-mile race. If you're training for a 10K, half marathon, or marathon, then race pace for you would be slower, depending on the race distance. For a faster runner (someone capable of doing a 5K in 15:00, for example), race pace would be much faster, near 5:00 per mile.

One side benefit of working out at race pace is that it gets you to recruit fast-twitch muscle fibers. According to Dr. Pate: "If those fibers have not been used in training, they may not be recruited easily when you get into a competitive situation."

Pace 2: Medium Intensity

Also important to training are lactate threshold runs. The lactate threshold in a trained runner would be 80 to 90 percent of his or her VO_2 max. Dr. Pate prescribes running longer but somewhat slower in Pace 2 workouts: 20 to 60 minutes at 70 to 90 percent of your MHR. "Not as fast as during an interval workout, but faster than the pace used on a long run," he instructs. In other words, set a pace *slower* than your 5K time. The runner capable of an 8:00 mile pace, for example, would do lactate threshold runs at about an 8:30 pace.

When Dr. Pate was training for the Boston Marathon (he had top-10 finishes there in 1975 and 1977), he would add a lactate threshold run to his Saturday routine as a prelude to his Sunday long runs.

He picked that workout intuitively. Later, as an exercise physiologist, he understood its scientific base. "Training studies have looked specifically at how to increase endurance performance," he says, "and some evidence suggests prolonged activity at intensities close to your current lactate threshold is helpful to increase that threshold."

Pace 3: Low Intensity

This is a longer run at a slower pace—a typical Saturday or Sunday morning workout for most serious runners. Many runners who are training for a marathon, for instance, choose 20 miles as the distance for their longest runs. In my 18-week marathon training programs, the longest run comes in

MEASURING YOUR MAX

Various training programs use maximum heart rate (MHR) as an aid to dictating workouts. Do you know yours?

The average person probably has an MHR somewhere around 200 beats a minute. But don't get too hung up on numbers, because people vary greatly depending on age and level of training. Also, various formulas used to predict MHR don't always work for everyone.

One formula is to take the number 220 and subtract your age. But *Aerobics* author Kenneth H. Cooper, MD, suggests that 200 minus half your age is more accurate for very fit people. That doesn't always work. At age 35, my predicted MHR should have been 185 using the first formula, 165 using the second. Actually, my MHR as measured at the Human Performance Laboratory at Ball State University was 160, suggesting the second formula as reasonably accurate. But for several decades as my age increased, my MHR declined very little.

On the other end of the scale, while coaching a high school cross-country team, I once placed a heart monitor on ninth-grader Megan during an interval workout. Megan's pulse jumped to 240 while running 400-meter reps on the track. I was ready to call 911, but that

Week 15, right before the 3-week taper. For most long runs, you should run aerobically, at a steady pace near 70 percent of your MHR. "Longer runs are valuable," says Dr. Pate, "even if you're not training for a marathon."

The pace used in low-intensity runs should be slow enough so that you can converse with your training partner. Some runners have dubbed

"Longer runs are valuable even if you're not training for a marathon."

this the talk test. (If you cannot talk with your partner, then you are running too fast.) In designing training programs for marathoners, I usually recommend doing the long runs 30 to 90 seconds (or more) slower than race pace. A runner capable of an 8-minute-mile pace in a 5K would run at an 8:45 to 9:30-mile pace (or slower) on long runs if training for a 5K, and still slower if training for a marathon.

heart rate actually was normal for her. She was a very fit athlete who later placed second in the state championships while leading her school to the team title. (Megan later attended Indiana University and now is a podiatrist based in Chicago.)

You can measure your pulse rate with some accuracy using a watch and, holding the vein in your wrist, counting pulse beats per minute. Or, you can purchase a pulse monitor to do the job for you. It is a fancy watch that continuously spits out numbers as you run. If you check your numbers at the end of a hard interval workout on the track or in the last few hundred meters of a 5K or 10K race, you'll probably come pretty close to determining your MHR.

For complete accuracy, you need to be tested on a treadmill at a performance laboratory. The standard stress test given by cardiologists during physical exams doesn't always produce the right number because cardiologists often are conservative and stop the treadmill before their patients reach maximum stress levels. For that reason, if you follow a training program by a coach that dictates workouts in percentages of max heart rate, you may need to interpret what that coach is telling you.

Pace 4: Rest

Can doing nothing be considered a pace? Well, yes. I consider rest equally important to all other workouts of the week. What is rest? Seems like a silly question, but I consider rest to be slow running at short distances or even a complete day off. "Some people do quite a lot of running on their recovery days," according to Dr. Pate, "but for others, any activity should be minimal. If they do too much on rest days, they either are going to get injured or they become so tired they need to back off on their hard days midweek, which defeats the purpose of the entire training plan."

Dr. Pate considers variety the key to any training program. He also subscribes to periodization, or peaking. "I continue to be attracted to the concept of building on intensity as one works toward achieving a major goal in some particular competition," he says. "There is risk associated with high-intensity exercise. Experience indicates that such workouts are more demanding and stressful. Carrying on high-frequency training for prolonged periods is risky in terms of overtraining and even riskier in terms of injury."

So to improve your speed endurance, surround your key sessions with sound recovery activities—such as short, easy runs; swimming; or walking. Cross-training, so to speak. Build your program on priorities. The highest priority is attached to the key hard sessions, so take the rest days when necessary to prevent breakdown and injury.

To vary the mix, I often prescribe cross-training on easy days, particularly for novice runners. Biking, swimming, or even walking can allow you to log some aerobic training while still resting the muscles specific to running. Don't make the mistake, however, of biking, swimming, or walking too hard or too much, or you'll defeat the purpose of the rest day.

CHAPTER NINE

JUGGLING WORKOUTS
Make the most of training time

f there is a single most frequently asked question on my various online forums, it certainly would be some variation of the Juggling Workout Theme: "Can I move my long run three weeks out from the marathon to four weeks out?" "What about two weeks out?" "Can I run my next speed-work session on Tuesday or Thursday instead of Wednesday?" "Is it okay to do my pace runs on Sundays and my long runs on Saturdays, instead of how you have them listed on your Web site?"

My answer usually is: *Yes!*

A lot of thought went into the training schedules in this book and online. I don't write workouts on slips of paper and pick them miscellaneously out of a jar. There is a method to my madness. I usually program long runs for the weekends, simply because people with 9-to-5 jobs have more spare time on weekends. I program rest days immediately before and immediately after those weekend running binges. In the middle of the week, I usually follow a hard day with an easy day, and follow an easy day with a hard day. There is a very definite pattern to my training programs. (The same can be said for the training programs of other coaches.)

A runner from Salt Lake City once asked me if he could do his long runs on Mondays instead of weekends. Yes, I responded. Schedules should not be followed mindlessly. Later, I used this example in lectures to illustrate that workouts can be juggled for convenience. My audiences often chuckle at this runner so nervous about making a seemingly meaningless change.

But in many respects, the Salt Lake City runner gets the last laugh. It *does* matter whether you do that long run on a Saturday, Sunday, or Monday. Which day you do your long run affects every other type of workout you do the rest of the week. Do your long run too close to a speed session, and your speedwork will suffer. Even worse, you could wind up injured.

Many runners do follow my programs precisely, taping a copy to the refrigerator, making a mark or writing a mileage number for every workout accomplished, right up to race day. They do this with pride and often post pictures of their workout sheet on Facebook. They show up at expos and ask me to autograph their completed sheets. I love that! The fact that they do follow the program precisely helps them build confidence for race day.

One runner who likes the refrigerator approach is Denise Feinen, 51, a business owner from Forestville, New York. Feinen followed one of my half marathon programs, "crossing the T's and dotting the I's." She says: "I was diligent to make sure I didn't change anything. It gave me confidence for my first half."

Control was one reason Ginny Owen, 58, an administrative assistant from Chambersburg, Pennsylvania, also decided to follow a training program for her first marathon. "I was more afraid of doing too much, out of enthusiasm, than not being able to run the miles," she says.

Yet many other runners, most often experienced runners, consider my programs guidelines rather than exact matrixes of workouts to be done exactly as written. Connie Ross Ciampanelli, 63, a high school guidance office secretary from North Providence, Rhode Island, says: "I follow the plan as closely as possible and daily check off each day's workout. I note anything special that happened and also mark what I do for cross-training on any particular day. I like the visual feedback I get illustrating my progress."

Yet Ciampanelli adds: "I don't have any problem juggling workouts. Life and weather sometimes get in the way."

How then do you balance long runs with speedwork? How do you mix easy runs, cross-training, and total rest? Those are some of the most difficult decisions made by coaches and runners. Get the formula right, and you set PRs. Get it wrong, and you become injured—or do less than your best.

THE SCIENCE OF TRAINING

Unfortunately, the scientific community offers little guidance. Russell H. Pate, PhD, of the University of South Carolina admits: "It's difficult to find funding for training-related issues, but it's also very difficult research to do. You're trying to control the behavior patterns of athletes who are not very inclined to be controlled."

Nevertheless, there are a few questions that runners need to ask when designing their own workout schedules or when modifying an existing training plan, like the ones in this book, to suit their work, family, and personal schedules. David E. Martin, PhD, of Georgia State University, a coach and consultant for the U.S. Olympic Committee, asks the following questions of the athletes he advises.

Recovery. How much rest do you need after your last workout? Muscle soreness, carbohydrate and fluid depletion, fatigue, and age all dictate how soon and how well you can do another hard run.

Rest. How much rest do you need before your next workout? You can't run well while suffering from the symptoms listed in Recovery. Resting before a hard workout allows you to train even harder and build more muscle.

Fitness. What shape are you in? Your current fitness level dictates not only how hard you can train-but also how quickly you recover. Very fit athletes can squeeze more hard runs into their workout weeks.

Schedule. What is your overall plan? Preset schedules are not meant to be followed precisely, but deviate too much and you may fail to achieve your goals.

Distraction. What's in your way? No matter how well-designed your training plan, distractions (the flu, a snowstorm, an important business engagement) may force you to make adjustments. (Interestingly, at least for elite athletes, Dr. Martin classifies a boyfriend or a girlfriend as a distraction.)

Fail to ask these questions, suggests Dr. Martin, and you'll never achieve success. Yet answer incorrectly, and you're also likely to struggle. Most critical when it comes to juggling workouts is how to mix hard days with easy days so that you recover to run hard again. According to Edward F. Coyle, PhD, a professor in the Department of Kinesiology and Health Education at the University of Texas at Austin, "Recovery is related to how long it takes you to refuel your muscles with glycogen. This becomes especially important if the intensity of exercise is high."

So which hard training sessions do you select and how much do you rest between them? In designing various training programs, I have relied frequently on the expertise of Dr. Pate. I recommend that you do likewise. He offers the following advice, which may be among the most important you will encounter in this book.

1. **Think recovery first.** Athletes do better when given adequate periods of recovery between extremely demanding exercise sessions. Know how much rest you need to retain quality in your schedule.

2. **Decide what's important.** Whether long runs for marathoners or speedwork for 5K runners, plug that most important "kingpin" workout into your schedule first.

3. **Build around the kingpin.** One or 2 other days a week, include other hard workouts to also build speed endurance. Marathoners might add long repeats at race pace (5 × 1 mile); 5K runners might include a medium-long run such as a 10-miler on the weekend.

4. **Fill in the gaps.** On the remaining days, add some low-stress running to contribute to your overall base mileage. Don't get hung up on numbers, but train consistently.

5. **Monitor body signals.** No coach can look inside your body. You need to recognize symptoms of overtraining or possible injury and make the necessary adjustments.

"The patterns are the same," advises Dr. Pate. "Only the specific training activities differ." Learn to juggle your workouts properly, and you are on your way to success in your next race.

PLOT YOUR PROGRAM

But how do you blend theory and reality? What can you learn from the eminent experts quoted in this book to help you run faster? Can the same training methods that permit American record holder and Olympic silver medalist Galen Rupp to run 10,000 meters in under 27 minutes work for someone whose goal is twice that length of time for the same distance? Yes, because regardless of your ability or performance potential, you can improve if you train correctly. If you learn how to blend hard work and easy work, fast running and slow running, all combined with adequate rest, you will run faster.

As we move forward structuring a program to develop speed endurance, keep in mind the principles covered so far. In the sample plan that follows, the particular distances you run will vary depending upon the race for which you are training. Someone training for a 5K would run shorter distances than someone training for a marathon, but that same 5K runner would also train at a faster relative pace. Consider the following training plan a suggestion that can be customized to your personal running goals. While my training programs are plentiful throughout this book, feel free to construct your own.

Note that the Pace entries relate to the various intensities described in Chapter 8's "Smart Training" section (see page 70). As a reminder, the four paces described there are Pace 1: High Intensity; Pace 2: Medium Intensity; Pace 3: Low Intensity; and Pace 4: Rest.

SUNDAY: LONG RUN

Distance: 10 to 20 miles

Intensity: Low

Pace 3: 30 to 90 seconds slower than race pace

Purpose: To strengthen aerobic base

MONDAY: RECOVERY

Distance: 0 to 6 miles

Intensity: Low

Pace 3: 30 to 90 seconds slower than race pace

Purpose: To recuperate from Sunday's long run

TUESDAY: SPEEDWORK

Distance: 3 to 6 miles

Intensity: High

Pace 1: Race pace (depending on race you are training for)

Purpose: To increase VO$_2$ max and efficiency

WEDNESDAY: RECOVERY

Distance: 3 to 6 miles

Intensity: Low

Pace 3: 30 to 90 seconds slower than race pace

Purpose: To recuperate from Tuesday's speedwork

THURSDAY: LACTATE THRESHOLD RUN

Distance: 5 to 10 miles

Intensity: Medium

Pace 2: 15 to 30 seconds slower than race pace

Purpose: To increase lactate threshold

FRIDAY: REST

Distance: 0 miles

Intensity: None

Pace 4: No running except for advanced runners

Purpose: To store energy for a weekend of hard work

SATURDAY: SWING DAY

Distance: 5 to 10 miles

Intensity: Medium to high

Pace 1 or 2: Race pace or slightly slower

Purpose: Competition or other fast training

Developing a training program is as much an art as a science. As we continue, we'll begin to discuss some of the increments that can be included in a training program to make you a faster and better runner. You will also learn how to use these guidelines as a matrix to develop training programs for various distances. I already have shown you three programs—novice, intermediate, advanced—designed for the 5K. In the next chapter, I'll modify those programs for a slightly longer distance, the 8K.

CHAPTER TEN

THE 8K

Training plans for this 'tween distance

While fact-checking this third edition of *Run Fast*, I texted my grandson Kyle Higdon. He was only 4 years old when the first edition was published in 1992, and he was a 12-year-old in middle school, just beginning to compete in cross-country and track, when the second edition was published in 2000. Now Kyle is a graduate student in aeronautical engineering at the University of Texas in Austin. In his spare time he coaches a local running club. Before that, he ran cross-country and track for the University of Notre Dame. I now find that I go to him for advice as much as he comes to me.

My question was simple: "Is 8K still the commonly run distance in college?" Despite the brevity of my text message, I knew that Kyle understood that I was talking about the men, rather than the women. (The men run the 8K followed by a climactic 10K at championships and women run 5K during the season followed by a 6K at late-season championship events such as the NCAA.)

Kyle responded quickly: "It seems like 8K races are rare other than college. I think there's maybe one in Austin."

Well, maybe there were still a few things I could teach my grandson. It is not every day I get a chance to one-up a rocket scientist. I texted back: "Shamrock Shuffle in Chicago. Over 22,000 runners."

Indeed, the Shamrock Shuffle is the largest 8K race in the United States with 22,873 finishers in 2015. No other 8K races are close in numbers, though three events each had around 10,000 finishers: Buffalo, New York; Madison, Wisconsin; and Virginia Beach, Virginia. The Autism Speaks 8K in Austin, mentioned by Kyle, attracted only a few hundred runners.

The Shamrock Shuffle attracts a large number of mostly Chicago-area runners because it signals the opening to the local running season. The Chicago Marathon, held later in the fall, will close it. When founded, the Shamrock Shuffle was held on the weekend nearest to St. Patrick's Day (thus the name), but got moved several weeks later into the spring to seek slightly better weather. After what invariably is a hard winter of snow, ice, and sleet, Chicago runners hop off their treadmills and flock to the outdoors as soon as the temperatures warm up and the sun comes out.

It became apparent to me one year that many of the participants in the Shamrock Shuffle were running newcomers. That year, despite the April date, temperatures spiked near 70 degrees. Many runners were overdressed, wearing winter running clothes that were soon soaked with sweat. When they left their homes several hours before the early-morning start, the temperature probably had been in the 40s, tempting them to dress as though it were still winter. A serious mistake, as they soon discovered. An experienced runner would probably not make that mistake.

Because I live around the bottom of the lake, a little more than an hour's drive from downtown Chicago, I like to consider the Shamrock Shuffle my hometown race. And a lot of runners prepare for the race using one of my 8K programs.

Why is a program necessary? Can't you just go out and run a few miles a few days of the week with maybe a slightly longer run on the weekends and be able to finish an 8K? Well, yes. But you didn't purchase *Run Fast* to be put off with such vague directions. You want to see improvement and achieve your goal. I want to help you achieve your goal. This is where a training program dedicated to the 8K comes into play.

Among the coaches and scientists I respect the most is Greg McMillan,

MS. He is a formidable presence on the Internet when it comes to providing instruction and training tips for runners. Most valuable among Greg's offerings are his prediction charts that allow runners to plug in a finish time and calculate an estimated pace for a given race distance, be it 5K, 8K, or marathon.

I asked McMillan why runners might need a dedicated 8K training program, and he offered this response that seems spot-on to me: "Training plans are designed to provide structure, accountability, and motivation. They build your physical and mental fitness from week to week, but remember that each athlete is an experiment of one. So, athletes must be open to modifying plans based on how they feel. The most successful athletes balance discipline and dedication with flexibility and openness to change. Ultimately, a smart training plan that fits within your ever-changing life is the one that will lead you to success."

With those remarks in mind, let's talk about the 8K, and how you are going to improve your PR at that distance. Or, if you have not run an 8K, how to establish a PR. First, how far is 8K? For those of you challenged metrically, 8 kilometers is just short of 5 miles: precisely 4.97097 miles. There is so little difference between 8K and 5 miles that a training program for an 8K event can be used for 5-mile races, although the mile distance is much less popular than the metric distance.

The 8K serves as an "in-between" distance, almost an "offbeat" distance occupying a position between the much more popular 5K and 10K distances. Could you use programs for those bookending distances to train for an 8K? Sure you could, but now that you have 8K programs for novice, intermediate, and advanced runners, you might as well use one of those.

What do the terms in each box within the tables mean? Seemingly, the answer to that question should be fairly obvious if you used one of my 5K programs, but here is a reminder. When asked to "run," do so at a comfortable, conversational pace. Cross-training should be aerobic: an easy bike ride, swimming, walking. More detailed definitions can be found in Chapter 3, and in the 5K Novice program, which can be found in Chapter 4.

HIGHER MILEAGE

The 8K Novice training plan features somewhat higher total mileage than the miles prescribed for runners doing a 5K. This is to be expected because the 8K event is somewhat farther than the 5K.

The 8K Novice

WEEK	MON	TUE	WED	THU	FRI	SAT	SUN
1	Rest or run/walk	2 mile run	30 min cross	2 mile run	Rest	30 min cross	2 mile run
2	Rest or run/walk	2 mile run	30 min cross	2 mile run	Rest	30 min cross	2.5 mile run
3	Rest or run/walk	2.5 mile run	35 min cross	2 mile run	Rest	40 min cross	3 mile run
4	Rest or run/walk	2.5 mile run	35 min cross	2 mile run	Rest	40 min cross	3.5 mile run
5	Rest or run/walk	2.5 mile run	40 min cross	2 mile run	Rest	50 min cross	4 mile run
6	Rest or run/walk	3 mile run	40 min cross	2 mile run	Rest	50 min cross	4 mile run
7	Rest or run/walk	3 mile run	45 min cross	2 mile run	Rest	60 min cross	4.5 mile run
8	Rest or run/walk	3 mile run	30 min cross	2 mile run	Rest	Rest	8K race

The 8K Intermediate schedule offers some speedwork on Wednesdays. I recommend alternating tempo runs with interval training. See Chapters 15 and 13, respectively, for detailed instructions on how to do those workouts. This intermediate plan includes runs on Mondays, unlike the equivalent 5K plan, which calls for a complete day off. It also features more miles on Tuesdays and Thursdays as compared with the 8K Novice plan. Be sure to rest on Fridays, and try to fit in an hour of cross-training on Saturdays. The Sunday runs peak at 7 miles, which is actually longer than race distance. Similar to my marathon training plans, I schedule stepback (slightly shorter) runs on Sundays for Weeks 3 and 6 to provide a small break from the mileage built up.

The 8K Advanced schedule features another (and final) step-up in difficulty. The main difference between this and the 8K Intermediate plan is

The 8K Intermediate

WEEK	MON	TUE	WED	THU	FRI	SAT	SUN
1	3 mile run	3 mile run	30 min tempo run	3 mile run	Rest	60 min cross	4 mile run
2	3 mile run	3.5 mile run	6 × 400 5K pace	4 mile run	Rest	60 min cross	5 mile run
3	3 mile run	4 mile run	35 min tempo run	3 mile run	Rest	60 min cross	3 mile run
4	3 mile run	4.5 mile run	7 × 400 5K pace	4 mile run	Rest	60 min cross	5 mile run
5	3 mile run	5.0 mile run	40 min tempo run	3 mile run	Rest	60 min cross	6 mile run
6	3 mile run	5.5 mile run	8 × 400 5K pace	4 mile run	Rest	60 min cross	4 mile run
7	3 mile run	6 mile run	45 min tempo run	3 mile run	Rest	60 min cross	7 mile run
8	3 mile run	3 mile run	4 × 400 5K pace	1-3 mile run	Rest	Rest	8K race

that there are two days of speedwork—and they are back-to-back on Tuesdays and Wednesdays. For advanced runners, that should not be a problem. You are "advanced," aren't you? Tempo runs on Tuesdays need not be hard. If you finish that workout exhausted, you miss the point of what a tempo run should be. The interval training on Wednesdays features repeats at mile pace, the pace you should be capable of running a 1500-meter or a mile race. Never run at those short distances? Use a performance chart, which you can easily find online, to determine an estimated pace that is based on a previous 5K or 10K time.

Saturday's workouts probably need some explanation: "4 mile total, 2 mile pace" means that you go for a 4-mile run with 2 miles in the middle being at your goal pace for 8K. Sunday's long runs are somewhat longer than in the intermediate program. In Week 5 of this advanced program, I suggest doing the 8 miles as a 3/1 workout. In other words, the first three-quarters of the run (6 miles) is at an easy pace, with the final quarter (2 miles) at a faster speed. As for the absence of any cross-training, I have found that advanced runners often do not have the patience to cross-train. They prefer to run, not fool around on a bicycle or swim in a pool. If you are more triathlon-oriented, feel free to program in some non-running workouts once or twice a week, most appropriately on easy days.

The 8K Advanced

WEEK	MON	TUE	WED	THU	FRI	SAT	SUN
1	3 mile run	30 min tempo run	6 × 400 mile pace	4 mile run	Rest or 3 mile run	4 mile total 2 mile pace	6 mile run
2	3 mile run	35 min tempo run	7 × 400 mile pace	5 mile run	Rest or 3 mile run	4 mile total 2 mile pace	7 mile run
3	3 mile run	40 min tempo run	5 × 400 mile pace	3 mile run	Rest or 3 mile run	5 mile total 2 mile pace	4 mile run
4	3 mile run	30 min tempo run	8 × 400 mile pace	5 mile run	Rest or 3 mile run	Rest	5K test
5	3 mile run	45 min tempo run	9 × 400 mile pace	6 mile run	Rest or 3 mile run	5 mile total 3 mile pace	8 mile run (3/1)
6	3 mile run	30 min tempo run	6 × 400 mile pace	3 mile run	Rest or 3 mile run	Rest	5K test
7	3 mile run	50 min tempo run	10 × 400 mile pace	6 mile run	Rest or 3 mile run	5 mile total 3 mile pace	8 mile run (3/1)
8	3 mile run	30 min tempo run	5 × 400 mile pace	3 mile run	Rest or 1-3 mile run	Rest	8K race

Please note that I have suggested test 5K races in Weeks 4 and 6 to get you in tune for the climactic 8K at the end of Week 8. Races at the 5K distance are very common, but if you can't find a 5K race on the weekend subscribed, don't worry. Any distance will do, and as an advanced runner you certainly can juggle workouts to accommodate these tests. No races at all? In my experience, a time trial over an accurately measured 3-mile or 5K course will keep me happy, although I always find it difficult to motivate myself to run anywhere near peak speed during a workout.

CHAPTER ELEVEN

GOOD FORM

Economy of motion is the ultimate weapon

While writing an article on American long-distance star Bob Kennedy for *Runner's World* magazine some time ago, I traveled to Indiana University in Bloomington and watched the two-time Olympian train on Old Kinser Pike, a country road south of the campus. I was struck by his technique.

While his legs and arms churned rapidly, Kennedy's torso did not move. From hips to head, he looked like a statue being towed along a rail. His body gleamed with sweat (the only symptom of the stress of running a near-5-minute-mile pace on a warm day), but his face was a mask. His eyes stared straight ahead. No smile. He seemed totally focused on the act of running as fast as he could.

Kennedy was running that day with Andy Herr, a training partner with 29:30 10K credentials, but Andy had to struggle to stay close. Kennedy and Herr had run the opening miles of an 8-mile workout over a series of imposing hills at a variety of paces. They were followed in a car by Sam Bell, the Indiana coach, who stopped the car each mile to call split times. As Kennedy cruised by the 4-mile mark, Bell shouted to him, "You're 20:21! This next mile is supposed to be hard."

"Hard" has different meanings to different people. Kennedy had been running lockstep to that point with Herr, but in shifting to a hard pace Kennedy moved effortlessly away.

Bell called out the next split: "4:19!"

Ummm, excuse me? For most runners, who might be hard-pressed to run even a half-mile in the time of 4:19, it's difficult to imagine the combination of talent and training that would result in a mile split—in practice, no less—that fast. Yet talent and training are only part of the picture. Much of Kennedy's ability to run fast came from his efficient running form. But was Kennedy's smooth stride a result of natural ability, or a result of practice-makes-perfect technique?

It probably was a combination of both.

PRACTICE MAKES PERFECT

A video of Kennedy winning the US national high school cross-country championship his senior year (claimed Coach Bell), showed that he ran smooth, though he was hunched over and wasted his energy with an up-and-down motion. While Kennedy was being coached by Bell as a student at Indiana University, those minor form faults disappeared. "My form definitely became more refined during my years at Indiana University," concedes Kennedy.

Talent and training are only part of the picture.

Good form is a skill that's sometimes overlooked when experts discuss what makes a top distance runner. We know that we need strong legs, a strong heart, and a strong mind in order to run fast. We also know that it helps to have only about 10 percent body fat. But one important factor that determines whether you finish near the front or rear of your local 5K race is an efficient running style, or effective biomechanics. In other words: good form.

We can change our form, but only to a certain point. An experienced coach can tell a runner how to incline his head, how to hold his arms, and how to land on—and push off with—his feet. In essence, how to look like a refined runner. "We spend a lot of time on body awareness," states Coach Bell. But coaching can only refine what Mother Nature gave you. Some of us are born with an efficient form, and some of us have to learn to live with what we have. We come from the womb preprogrammed for success or failure as runners, the biomechanical relationship of arms to legs to trunk already determined.

Nevertheless, even inefficient runners can improve. David L. Costill, PhD, remembers the time when three girls from one family, the Cartwrights, began running local road races. "When they started," recalls Dr. Costill, "they finished behind me, but as they got older, they gradually moved past." At age 13, Lora Cartwright, the oldest, set an age-group record of 2:55:00 in the marathon. She won several state championships and later competed for Purdue University.

Dr. Costill continues, "The most noticeable thing from year to year was that they began as bouncers, because that's the way kids run. The older they got and the more they ran, the smoother they got. Exercise physiologist Jack Daniels, PhD, did some research in which he followed elementary and junior high school kids at 6-month intervals, measuring their oxygen uptake while they ran at a set speed. What he learned was that as they got older, their VO_2 max didn't change. What happened was that they became more efficient. As a result, their times got faster. These improvements seem to be natural in young, developing kids, so the big question is: How do you help older runners improve their form?"

Dr. Costill believes that motor patterns developed early in life become "frozen." While subtle adjustments can be made in those motor patterns to improve performance, major changes will not occur. This is particularly true in Dr. Costill's primary sport of swimming. "You learn a smooth stroke early," he believes, "or you never learn." He also cites speech patterns, because they, too, become locked in place early. I have four cousins, for example, who emigrated from Italy to the United States at various ages, from 6 to 26. Their accents are related to the ages at which they arrived. Nearly a half-century later, the youngest sounds typically American; the oldest sounds like he just arrived. Speech therapy and study can help people improve their speech patterns, but some accents never fade.

Similarly, running-stride patterns may also resist improvement. An economical form is not achieved easily. Some experts even insist that it happens naturally, that it should not be taught. Some of the greatest runners in history have nontraditional running forms that seem inefficient to spectators, but race results prove otherwise. Emil Zatopek had terrible upper-body form, yet he was arguably among the greatest distance runners of all time, winning the 5000, 10,000, and marathon "triple" in the 1952 Olympic Games. Alberto Salazar was known for his unique running form, yet he set a world marathon record. Paula Radcliffe, the British runner and Olympian who set the world marathon record of 2:15:25 at the 2003 London Marathon—an incredible achievement that still stands as of the printing of this book—has one of the oddest running forms in the sport.

"People run as they do because they have to," one college coach told me. "They don't have any choice. A lot of time is spent coaching things you don't have to, and this is one of them."

Yet Coach Bell took exception to that statement when I repeated it to him. "What he's saying is that you can't coach," countered Bell. "I happen to disagree with that."

Can your natural style or form be changed? How can you learn to run economically?

POSITIVE GAINS

You can make your style somewhat more economical, even if you started running as an adult. Joanne Kittel is a perfect example. When she joined a beginning running class I taught, Kittel was not the world's least economical runner, but she was close.

At one time, Kittel weighed 196 pounds. Over a period of years, before joining my class, she lost 80 pounds. So she at least looked like a runner—that is, when she was standing still. Kittel ran bent over, almost stumbling, gasping for breath sometimes. I was afraid to correct her running form for fear that any distraction would send her tumbling to the ground.

Kittel, however, persevered. She became every coach's dream—a runner with the desire to improve. Gradually, she built her running base. She went from slogging through 1 or 2 miles to covering 3 or 4 miles without tripping over a crack in the pavement. At classes and clinics, she paid attention when much swifter runners talked about speedwork. Soon, Kittel was doing early-morning strides on the same golf course fairway where I often trained. Later, she did some interval training by making one-quarter-mile marks on a flat stretch of road that paralleled some railroad tracks. I taught her a few of these tricks, but mostly she learned by listening to others.

One morning, I was working in my office. I glanced out the window and saw this fast female striding smoothly past. It was Kittel! I remembered the stumbling woman who had seemed so uncoordinated when I first saw her in my class, and I was amazed. Eventually, Kittel would run 3:45:00 for the marathon, nowhere near as fast as Radcliffe, but a solid performance that many runners would be proud to achieve. For me, her accomplishments confirmed Coach Bell's philosophy that running economy can be a learnable trait, and that it is not merely a gift of genetics.

LESS IS MORE

But exactly what is an economical runner? Owen Anderson, PhD, an exercise scientist and former columnist for *Runner's World*, discussed the subject of economy in an article for a newsletter he edited, *Running Research News:* "An economical runner is one who burns modest amounts of oxygen at a given pace; an uneconomical runner requires large amounts of oxygen (and energy) for the same running speed." In other words, if you are an economical runner when you're running at the same speed as your competitors, the pace feels easier to you than it does to them. Put another way, when you're running with the same effort as your competitors, you're running faster than they are.

Dr. Anderson believes, as I do, that running economy is a neglected aspect of training. He indicated that while exercise physiologists seemingly have solved the secrets of boosting VO_2 max to create faster runners, little is known about which training methods best improve running economy, the skill that often separates good runners from bad.

Martyn Shorten, a professor from Loughborough University in Great

Running economy is a neglected aspect of training.

Britain, admits that trying to turn inefficient runners into smooth striders is not easy. He suggests two possibile targets.

Flexibility. First, lack of flexibility restricts range of movement and may limit economy. Thus, runners interested in improving their form should first improve their flexibility. This is why so many coaches stress stretching drills, a subject covered in Chapter 17 (starting on page 189).

Smoothness. Second, Shorten added that jerky movements incur an energy cost without contributing to efficient propulsion. "In coach's terms," he summarized, "an efficient running action will appear to be smooth, relaxed, and rangy—but you don't need a computer to tell you that." Converting jerky movements into smooth movements is no easy task, but it's one that sometimes can be accomplished with the use of speed drills, also covered in Chapter 17 (see "Flexibility Drills That Build Speed" on page 198).

One of the smoothest runners I competed against was Curt Stone. Stone attended Pennsylvania State University and later competed for the New York Athletic Club. He was America's premier distance runner when I first became involved in track and field. He placed sixth in the 1948 Olympic 5000 meters. I was still in high school then, but 4 years later, I ran against him at the 1952 Olympic Trials in California, where he won the 10,000 and set an American record. A week later, I watched at the Los Angeles Coliseum as he won the 5000 meters in the Trials and set another American record.

Of all the dozen or so runners on the Coliseum track that day, Stone easily was the smoothest. He moved along the surface with minimum effort, his inevitable triumph seemingly preordained by his ability, whether practiced or God-given, to run with economy of style. Of course, Stone didn't win every race—no runner does. In fact, at the 1952 Olympics in Helsinki, he lost decisively to Zatopek—the man who moved like a maniac. Even then, I continued to admire Stone for his economy of motion.

But my story does not end there. A half-dozen years later, at a meet in which I ran well, a track aficionado approached me and asked, "Do you know who you look like when you run?" I replied, "Who?" To my surprise, he said, "Curt Stone!"

Did I run like Stone because, after that day in the Coliseum, I modeled my running after his? Or did I merely think he ran better because I had already realized, at least subconsciously, that I ran like him?

SHORT STRIDES, FAST FINISH

I recall another runner from my past: Jim Beatty, one of the world's best milers and 5000-meter runners in the early 1960s, and later a TV commentator. Beatty is now a member of the USA Track and Field (USATF) Hall of Fame. But in 1956, the two of us were unheralded members of an American track team that spent 3 weeks training and competing in Finland. During a workout one afternoon at Suomen Urheilupisto, a sports camp near the town of Vierumaki, Finnish coach Armas Valste watched Beatty run an interval workout. Beatty was relatively short and stocky, but he had a long, flowing stride that allowed him to swallow long stretches of ground in large gulps. Valste observed him and commented tersely, "He overstrides!"

At the time, Beatty was still attending the University of North Carolina and had a mile best of about 4:07. He graduated and retired from the sport. Then, while watching the U.S.–Soviet track meet on television a few years later, he wondered how good he could become if he fully dedicated himself to excellence. He moved to Los Angeles to train under Mihaly Igloi, the former Hungarian Olympic coach who had defected to the United States in 1956. Igloi placed Beatty on a twice-daily, 100-mile-a-week program that consisted almost entirely of interval work on the track.

I next saw Beatty in 1959 during the telecast of an indoor mile race, and my first reaction was that he had cut his stride length in half. In actuality, Beatty probably had sliced only inches from it, but it appeared to be a short, quick-tempo, efficient running style that was well-suited to his height. He employed this short stride for maybe 10 of the 11 laps that made up the mile race. Then, almost as though he had shifted gears, he began a powerful, long-striding sprint that swept him past his opponents. He won that day in 3:59, a considerable improvement over his college time—and in an era when sub-4-minute miles remained a rarity.

Beatty had shown me that you can improve your running form to make it more efficient. Whether this improvement had come from a conscious manipulation of style by his coach or from an unconscious reaction by Beatty's body for protection during an exhausting training regimen, I don't know. His shift mirrored my own experience in seeing my stride shorten as I went from 25 miles a week in college to 100 miles a week several years later.

FIVE ELEMENTS OF EFFICIENT FORM

So what is good running form? And how do you recognize it? The two-time Olympian Fred Wilt, a contemporary of Stone, made an interesting analysis of running form in his book *The Complete Canadian Runner,* produced for the Canadian Track and Field Association. Some of Coach Wilt's views are included in this list of elements of form and how efficient runners use them. Read the following points, then ask yourself: "How do I stack up?"

You can improve your running form to make it more efficient.

Footstrike. The majority of better runners land on their midfoot; that is, at a point just behind the ball of the foot. They then drop down on their heel, and their body glides above the foot that is planted firmly on the ground before they push off with the toes. Some land more forward on the ball of the foot (toe runners); others land more flatfooted (heel strikers). Different runners have different plants, dictated by how the parts of their bodies fit together, otherwise known as biomechanics.

If you possess an imperfect footplant, if your foot pronates too much or too little (which can cause injury), you may need to see a podiatrist for orthotic inserts. Most runners, however, can control such problems by carefully selecting shoes. The worst thing you can do to your footstrike is to try to adjust your landing to accommodate what you think other runners do.

Stride length. There is no definition of a perfect stride length; the best stride lengths depend on each runner's natural form. In general, however, a short, quick-tempo stride may be more economical in a 5K or 10K race. A long stride causes the runner to lose momentum and waste energy by pushing too far ahead of his center of gravity—thus, the term *overstriding*. But understriding can be just as great a mistake. Attempting to manipulate your stride, based

TEACHING FORM

What allows Olympian Bob Kennedy to run so effortlessly? Coach Sam Bell describes Kennedy's form, a form he demanded of all his runners when he coached at Indiana University: "Bob runs tall. He wastes little energy. His head is parallel to the ground as he stares off into the distance. His back is straight, and his arms churn easily forward and back. As his arms come forward, they bend slightly as the relaxed hands (thumb resting on index finger) come to chest level.

"As the arms return backward, they straighten somewhat as the hand reaches back to the hip. Torso and head remain perpendicular to the ground. The whole body is relaxed."

How did Bell's runners achieve such form? Coach Bell emphasized acceleration sprints, body coordination drills, and relaxation sprints.

Acceleration sprints are simple: Runners start their 50-meter dash easily, progressively increasing to near-top speed, before jogging back to begin again. They concentrate on relaxation.

Coordination drills include a series of exercises. In one called High Knees, each runner runs in an exaggerated style, raising knees to waist height on each step. They also Skip for Distance, gliding forward while swinging arms to shoulder height.

Heel-to-glute drills emphasize quick, high backward kicks, the runner's heel hitting his butt with each stride. Several sidestepping moves complete the routine.

Bell next has his runners run a series of relaxation sprints "loose as a goose." Arm and leg movements are exaggerated as runners lope along as fast as possible, as though running on air or skimming across water, with each movement relaxed and light.

Eventually, the runner is shaped into an efficient and economical machine. Kennedy says, "Coach Bell told me that when finishing a race, you don't think, 'faster, faster, faster,' you think, 'form, form, form!' You relax, keep your form, and all of a sudden, speed comes."

on some article you read online, also poses risks. Experts suggest we should all aspire to 180 steps per minute, but athletes differ greatly when it comes to cadence. In tests at the Nike Sport Research Lab, laboratory director E. C. Frederick, PhD, measured my stride rate at between 192 and 196. Olympic marathon champion Joan Benoit Samuelson, tested at the same time (see the following page), exhibited a 200 cadence. *Running Times* author Phil Latter notes that Ethiopia's Kenenisa Bekele, a world record holder, ramped his stride rate up to 215 in the last lap while winning the 10,000 at the World Championships. Although 180 strides per minute is promoted by some experts as the perfect cadence, different runners may achieve success with different counts.

Carriage. Your trunk should be more or less perpendicular to the ground and your hips should be forward. American Olympian Garry Bjorklund once told me, "Novice runners have a tendency to sit down, to put their weight behind them. They need to bring their center of gravity forward and get their weight over their metatarsals (the part of your foot between the ankle and the toes)."

Arm carry. Your arms should move in rhythm with your legs. They should swing forward more than sideways, with your elbows in and your hands cupped (rather than clenched). The late Bill Bowerman, who was track coach for the University of Oregon, liked to have his runners carry their arms high across the chest. Villanova University's Jim "Jumbo" Elliott wanted his runners to carry their arms low, "thumbs in their pockets." If these two renowned coaches can differ as to what is proper form, then there may be no proper form.

Head position. The head serves as the keystone for the rest of the body. Back in some Paleolithic era, a coach once told me to fix my gaze 10 yards up the track and use my eyes to anchor my head in a relaxed position. That is probably as good advice as any. If you allow your eyes and gaze to wander all over the road, you probably will wander with them.

HIDDEN FORM FLAWS

I wonder how much even the most experienced coach can learn about a runner's form merely by observing with the naked eye. At the Nike Sport

Research Lab, I observed Joan Benoit Samuelson running on the treadmill. From the side, her legs seemed a blur as she ran at a 6-minute pace. I could tell little by observing her from different angles. She seemed to move very smoothly, another Curt Stone.

Yet Dr. Frederick pointed out that Samuelson favored her right leg, the result of a fracture while skiing years before. He knew this because they had analyzed her style by camera and computer. That analysis was 3 years before Samuelson strode into history with her victory in the first Olympic marathon for women, at Los Angeles in 1984. But it also was 3 years before a severe knee injury, perhaps caused by the imbalance detected by Dr. Frederick, forced her to have surgery that almost caused her to miss the Olympics.

Dr. Frederick told me that when they test various individuals, they sometimes discover that runners who appear to have the worst form are judged most efficient in the laboratory. By now it is common knowledge, for example, that four-time Boston and New York City Marathon champion Bill Rodgers, for all of his other virtues, had a strange right arm swing that compensates for a slight foot imbalance. And Frank Shorter swung his left arm outward. You wouldn't have wanted to pass him on that side for fear of getting struck. Dr. Frederick said that Tony Sandoval, winner of the 1980 Olympic Trials marathon, functioned like two separate runners in the area of footstrike: flatfooted on the left, a classic mid-footstrike on the right.

Woe to the coach who would have attempted to modify their forms. In the closing stages of a race, they moved with relentless energy and efficiency.

During another project, the scientists at the Nike Sport Research Lab tested footstrikes by having a group of top runners adjust their forms during different runs on the treadmill—one time landing on the balls of their feet, another time midfoot, another time more flatfooted, and even on their heels. They expected to discover that the midfoot landing was most efficient, since film and force plate analysis suggests that the world's fastest runners run that way.

In the tests, most of the runners found landing on their heels to be least comfortable. One subject described heel running during the test as a truly horrible experience. Yet when the results were computed, heel running proved the most efficient, even for that one reluctant subject. "Sometimes the more you learn, the more you realize how little you know," Dr. Frederick admits. He cautioned runners against using this one experiment to justify a major shift in their running style. "There may be other reasons, beyond what we can measure easily in a laboratory, why a runner should stick with a particular style," he warns. Despite scientific analysis, the best running form is the one that allows you to run quickly, efficiently, and injury free.

CREATING FORM AWARENESS

Let me offer not necessarily a magic formula but rather some suggestions as to how you might at least be aware of your running form, if not improve it. In his article in *Running Research News,* Dr. Anderson quoted several techniques used by Dr. Daniels to improve running form: interval training, downhill running, uphill running, and bounding drills. Each of these techniques are discussed in detail elsewhere in this book. But for now, let's briefly discuss how to use these drills to enhance your form.

Interval training has been proven as a way of improving running ability. It can strengthen you aerobically and anaerobically. It can strengthen your legs. It can strengthen your confidence. I've always felt that, for me, one of the greatest values of interval training is that it strengthened my ability to concentrate. It permitted me to maintain good form. During interval sessions at the beginning of the season, I would often find my mind drifting and my form lagging in the backstretch. As weeks went on and I became more comfortable with the training routine, I found I could concentrate and maintain an efficient form for the full lap. Maintaining peak efficiency over a longer period of time inevitably helped me to run faster. My times improved not merely in workouts but also in races.

Dr. Daniels apparently agrees, which suggests to Dr. Anderson that runners should combine short bouts of 400 meters, carried out at a rapid (but not maximum) velocity, with maximum rest: a work-to-rest ratio of 1 to 4 or greater. That is, for each quarter-mile you run in 75 seconds, you should rest

5 minutes or more. "The idea is to be completely rested and refreshed for every 400-meter run," Dr. Anderson says, "so that you can maintain good running form throughout."

Dr. Daniels also recommends downhill running as a technique for becoming accustomed to running faster by increasing your leg turnover without increasing your effort. He suggests running very gradual down-hills—no more than 2 percent grade. Golf course fairways are ideal. Uphill running, on the other hand, is good for improving the power of your butt muscles, getting them more involved in the motion of running and forcing you to use more effort. "The idea is not to sprint, but to move steadily," Dr. Daniels says.

You need to become aware of how your body moves as you run.

Bounding drills, championed by Coach Bell, similarly improve strength, flexibility, and running form.

Apart from what the experts say, I'm convinced that runners need to develop what Bell calls body awareness and what I call a feel for form. You need to become aware of how your body moves as you run. One way of achieving that is to attend a running camp or clinic where you can be filmed, so that you can see what you look like running. Many specialty running stores can film you running on a treadmill. Or, you can use a smartphone or camera on a video setting and have someone else record you.

To improve your running economy, try these form drills.

Run barefoot in the park. On a summer day, go to the beach or golf course and find a smooth stretch of sand or fairway. Remove your shoes. Jog or run at a comfortable pace for a distance of 50 to 100 meters. Can you feel the point where your foot contacts the ground? Do you land midfoot or more toward your toe or heel? Can you run more comfortably by adjusting your footstrike? Probably not, but at least you will be aware of your landing. Running gently on the grass is one way to develop body awareness. Running on wet sand and studying your footprints is another way.

Run fast at the track. Visit a 400-meter track. Begin running at the 300-meter starting line, at the head of the back straightaway. Slowly accelerate throughout that straightaway until you are running near race pace through the turn. As you come into the home straightaway, continue your acceleration so that you reach top speed by the time you reach the finish line. What happens to your form during this acceleration run? At what point and pace do you become a more efficient or less efficient runner?

10 TIPS ON RUNNING FORM

Fred Wilt was a distance runner on the 1948 and 1952 U.S. Olympic teams and became famous for his legendary indoor mile encounters with Wisconsin's Don Gehrmann. After retiring from the FBI, Wilt coached the women's running teams at Purdue University. He edited the publication *Track Technique* and advised various runners, including 1964 Olympian Buddy Edelen, who once held the world marathon record of 2:14:28. (Wilt also coached me when I achieved my PR at the Boston Marathon that same year.) The following is excerpted from a book Wilt produced for the Canadian Track and Field Association, *The Complete Canadian Runner.*

1. Running form is a completely individual issue. Each athlete differs from every other at least to a minute extent in height, weight, bone structure, length and size of muscles, point of muscle origin and insertion, strength, flexibility, posture, and personality, in addition to numerous other features. Therefore, no two runners should ever use identical form, even though they all adhere to basic mechanical principles.

2. It is a form error of the highest magnitude to run without permitting the heel to touch and rest on the ground with each stride, without reservation, in a ball-heel grounding action. This is true at all running speeds, especially sprinting.

3. It is physically possible to land heel-first in running, but this is quite incorrect and almost never seen, since it jars the body excessively and can be done only at very slow running speeds. Landing heel-first and "toe running" (refusing to permit the heels to ground) are both incorrect.

Focus on what happens to your knee lift, your stride length, your posture, your arm carry, and your head angle. At what point does fatigue cause your running form to deteriorate?

Run straight on the road. Pick a lightly trafficked road where you can follow a straight line: a painted stripe, a crack in the pavement, or the

4. Ideally, the position of the feet in running is one in which the inner borders fall approximately along a straight line. Athletes should run in a straight line, but not necessarily on such a line. When one foot is placed directly in front of the other, lateral (sideways) balance is impaired.

5. Runners in races longer than sprint distances wherein economy of energy is the paramount consideration should use a natural stride: not exaggerated, not long, not short, but of a length in keeping with maximum economy of effort for the running speed required.

6. Both understriding and overstriding are faults. Each runner has his own optimum stride length at any given speed, depending upon leg length, muscular strength, and joint flexibility.

7. At uniform top speed with zero acceleration, if the athlete was running in a vacuum with no wind resistance, there would be no body lean at all.

8. The hands should be carried in a relaxed, cupped position at all running speeds. They should never be rigidly clenched in a fist while running, since this produces tension, which causes unnecessary fatigue.

9. The head should be aligned naturally with the trunk, and the eyes should be focused a few meters ahead while running.

10. Usually, the best solution to apparent form problems is many repetitions of running short distances, such as 100 meters, at a fast, though not exhausting, pace.

separation between pavement and shoulder. Run at a steady race pace for 1 mile or more. Focus your attention on that line and think of yourself as a machine moving along it, like a train on a rail. Be a Buddha, like Bob Kennedy. Can you run straight along the line without wavering back and forth? Is your head straight; are your eyes level? Are your arms moving smoothly back and forth, in rhythm with your legs? Are your legs moving straight forward and kicking straight back?

Run focused in a race. As you're running your next 5K, try to concentrate completely on your movements. Can you ignore the scenery, the sights and sounds of the race around you? Can you run without talking? As for music playing through earbuds, forget it! Are you only peripherally aware of other runners around you? Can you maintain the form you practiced on the grass, on the track, on the road? You may need to do so if you want to maximize your ability to run fast.

CHAPTER TWELVE

THE SCIENCE OF SPEEDWORK

Fine-tune your training

"There's only one way to get faster," Olympian Francie Larrieu Smith told me. "You have to teach your legs what it feels like to run fast." Larrieu Smith recommends some sort of speedwork, whether repeats, intervals, fartlek, or whatever. She concedes that runners can improve their times by slowly conditioning themselves—the same pace, day after day. But eventually, improvement ceases. Runners hit a plateau. That's when speed-work can help.

It worked for Larrieu Smith. Between 1972 and 1992, she made five Olympic teams at distances between 1500 meters and the marathon, her best finish being fifth in the 10,000 meters in Seoul, Korea, with a time of 31:35:52. She went on to set 13 world indoor records and 35 United States records. She ran a 2:28:01 and placed second at the 1990 London Marathon. At the 1992 Olympics in Barcelona, Spain, she carried the United States flag into the stadium at the opening ceremony. An extraordinary athlete!

You would do well to listen to what Larrieu Smith says when she tells you to add speedwork to your regular training routine. Just try it and see if it helps you run faster.

Alas, a lot of runners are like one individual who came up to my booth one year at the Chicago Marathon expo. He fingered an early edition of *Run Fast* on the table, frowned, then looked up at me: "I don't want to run fast." Possibly that individual felt threatened by the type of training my book might ask him to do. A trio of older runners at another expo told me that they had a conversation one day and decided they didn't want to try any more training tricks. They felt that by sticking to their usual regimen they would be less likely to get injured. And they might be right. But I also remember Allison Wolf, one of the runners on the high school cross-country team I coached for a while in Michigan City. She once stated that she did not have the speed for running speedwork. I eventually convinced her otherwise, and she finished her high school career as captain of the team. I might also add that two dec-

Speedwork consists of any training done at race pace or faster.

ades later she was still running marathons, her best at Chicago, 3:14:59, well below the strict Boston Marathon qualifying standards.

HOW FAST IS SPEEDWORK?

What is speedwork? Different coaches might define speedwork differently. Because you have my book in hand, let me offer my definition: Speedwork consists of any training done at race pace or faster. This definition allows for variation in abilities. But which race do you use to define race pace? During the course of a year, I may compete at distances from 800 meters to a marathon. In college, I sometimes even ran a leg on the mile relay team. While my range is greater than that of many competitive runners, it is not unheard of. Take Larrieu Smith as one example, competing in the Olympics at races from the 1500 meters to the marathon.

Olympic champion Frank Shorter relates race pace to his average speed in a 2-mile run. During the period when Shorter ranked as one of the world's top 10,000-meter runners, he would consider speedwork as running faster than 65 seconds for a 400. A number of coaches tie speedwork to the 10K because it's a popular race distance and most runners can easily relate to it. Toward the end of my career as a masters runner and when my 5K times hovered around 25 minutes (8-minute-mile pace), my speedwork began around 2 minutes for a 400. As a younger runner, my speedwork time was closer to 1 minute for a 400. You don't want to hear where that speedwork time might be now. The most important point is that there is no single number; it differs for all of us.

Choose your pace carefully. A common beginner's mistake is to run speedwork flat out—faster than race pace. While a certain amount of flat-out training can contribute to your fitness level, too much of it can increase your risk of injuries.

MAKING SPEEDWORK FUN

A lot of runners do want to run fast, but remain unconvinced that they have either the ability or the determination to follow the advice of experts such as Larrieu Smith, or to follow the path of someone like Joanne Kittel (see page 92 for Kittel's story).

As a member of our local running club, Kittel once told me how much she despised speedwork. "Does it ever become fun?" she asked.

Fun: Why does speedwork have to be fun? I had no ready answer for Kittel. I find speedwork fun, maybe even exhilarating on occasion. Sure, I enjoy long runs on a path through the woods or along backcountry roads— but there also are times when I want to get out on an ugly asphalt track with no trees nearby and parched grass on the infield and simply pound away. Is this being masochistic? Possibly so.

Even elite runners who average more than 100 miles a week in their training concede that quality is more important than quantity. They know that you can't abandon speedwork in favor of so-called junk miles. Long runs on the roads and in the woods (whether you want to call them junk miles or not) do have their place in any runner's training plan, but not if it causes the abandonment of other forms of training.

During our discussion about speedwork, Kittel told me about the sort of speedwork she did. For one workout, she had marked a nearby road in quarter-mile increments. Running over this marked road, she would

Fun: Why does speedwork have to be fun?

alternate going fast and slow. Fast, slow. Fast, slow. Fast, slow. You can do the same. Push yourself to the point where you are breathing hard, then ease back on the throttle until you are breathing easy, then pick up the pace again. Kittel's workout reminded me of some of the workouts of Czech running star and multiple Olympic champion Emil Zatopek, who would use telephone poles as guideposts for his sprints, sometimes also seeing how many poles he could pass while holding his breath. Such speedwork could hardly be classified as fun.

A second workout Kittel used was to go to a nearby golf course and do sprints of 130 yards, jogging and walking in between. I doubt if she knew much about Zatopek's training, but I recognized the source of inspiration for that second workout. It was my own method. I often described it at my clinics. Why did we both use 130 yards? Because that was the distance from one tree to another on a particularly flat fairway where I trained. Kittel probably was using the same trees to mark her start and finish lines.

I enjoyed that particular golf course workout, because I rarely pushed it. Mine were strides rather than sprints, and there is a subtle difference, which you will learn in Chapter 16 (see page 177). I ran fast but seldom did so many repetitions that I finished tired. Typically, I ran a set of four to eight sprints or strides, jogging between, then I walked to full recovery. When I was in top shape, I would do a second set of eight. Why sets of eight? Why not? Good training is often as much an art as a science.

Does such a workout sound difficult or excessively painful to you? With those sprints done only slightly faster than race pace, and following a thorough warmup, would they be likely to cause more injury than a long run on the road? I don't think so. Done in the cool early morning at sunrise in the bucolic setting of a golf course, would the workout lack beauty? Again, I don't think so. And I believe that if you incorporate only this one workout into your training program for at least a few months during the summer, you will see an improvement in your performances.

Like many fast runners of my era, I came to road running with a track background. I competed in the mile and half-mile while at Carleton College in Northfield, Minnesota, and won conference titles in both those events. To me, speedwork seemed natural. But it could hardly seem so to Kittel, who came to one of my running classes as your classic beginning jogger. Like most runners who are more involved with personal achievement than with Olympic aspirations, she began by running slowly and progressed to running long then shifted to running short, which allowed her to run fast. Speedwork, therefore, was unnatural to her. It was a beast to be conquered.

So, it was not fun for Kittel. What was fun, however, was her 44:23 10K finish several weeks before our conversation. It was her first 10K run faster than 45 minutes. And to what did she attribute the improvement?

Speedwork!

Kittel would continue to mix fast running with her long training, whether she liked it or not. What she did like was the result of doing speedwork: fast race times. Speedwork may not have been the only reason—or even the major reason—for her success. Over a period of years, she had also built a base of miles and adjusted her running form, which contributed to her improvement. But speedwork certainly helped her break 45 minutes for the 10K. It can help you become a better runner too.

ACCEPT THE CHALLENGE

Before you begin to add speedwork to your training, you should consider whether you are ready to accept this challenge. Coach Bob Glover of the New York Road Runners recommends that runners not use speed training until they train for a full year, complete at least one competitive road race, average at least 16 miles per week running, and race faster than their training pace at distances between 3 and 6 miles.

"Be careful about how quickly you add speed training to your schedule," warns Bob Williams, a coach from Portland, Oregon. "Don't jump too rapidly from the base phase of your training program to two or three speed sessions a week. Many so-called overtraining injuries are simply the result of too much intensity too soon."

You should also be willing to push into the discomfort zone. I dislike using the word "pain," which has a negative connotation. I also find it difficult to understand why marathoners, who willingly suffer the agonies accompanying the last 6 miles of their race, are unwilling to accept what they consider to be painful sensations associated with speedwork. If you want to be a fast runner, you must be willing to accept a certain amount of discomfort. That doesn't mean speedwork is all discomfort. Integrated rest intervals act as a counterbalance. Just as quickly as you enter the discomfort zone, you leave it again by walking or jogging.

WHY SPEED TRAINING WORKS

There are several very important physiological reasons why speedwork is necessary if you want to maximize your potential at any distance, from the mile to the marathon. You have been waiting for me to offer you a sound reason to do speedwork, and here it is from Ball State physiologist William Fink. The primary reason, says Fink, is that you need to train your system to recruit the muscle fibers necessary to be able to run fast. "I must admit, a lot of the evidence is still out," suggests Fink, "but obtaining a sense of relaxation at race pace apparently comes as a result of training your muscle fibers to function at that accelerated pace."

But certain metabolic adaptations also occur, Fink explains, that relate to the pH levels of the muscles. When you run at an anaerobic level—that is, at a pace so fast you cannot absorb oxygen fast enough to eliminate your body's developing waste products—your muscles accumulate lactic acid. Your pH level declines. Eventually, so much lactic acid accumulates in your muscles that they lose their ability to contract. This is why a middle-distance runner who sprints a 400-meter race usually crosses the finish line stiff-legged, in a state of near collapse. His muscles (at least temporarily) no longer function properly because of excessive lactic acid. Although the phenomenon occurs over a much longer period of time, the same happens to someone running an all-out 5K or 10K.

Training, and particularly speed training, can modify this effect. According to Fink, "One of the adaptations is the development of a 'buffering' capacity on the part of the body. A runner who is well-trained, through use of the proper amounts of speedwork, can limit the degree to which his muscles become acidic. He can run faster for a longer time before accumulation of lactic acid brings him to a halt."

Also part of the training process is the psychological ability to continue to perform under high stress; in effect, to push on through the pain barrier. *Runner's World* columnist and speaker John Bingham talks about having the courage to start, but for success as a runner you also need the courage to continue, and the courage to push through the pain barrier. But a lot of what many runners, including beginners, assume to be psychological adaptations may actually be metabolic ones—particularly pushing back the anaerobic threshold.

In the words of the late physiologist Al Claremont, PhD, "Too many people write themselves off as having bad bodies, when they possess more potential than they realize. They simply are unwilling to do the hard work, including speed training, necessary to convert their supposed bad body into a good one."

The anaerobic threshold for someone with "poor" ability might be 50 or 60 percent of maximum; that is, they might begin to accumulate lactic acid in their muscles while running at near half their MHR. For an "average" runner, it could be 70 percent, and a "good" runner may still be able to function aerobically at 85 percent of maximum. Speed-trained runners push into the world beyond. This level of conditioning permits the fastest runners to run seemingly endless miles below a 5-minute pace without apparent distress, because lactic acid has not yet started to accumulate.

For success as a runner you need the courage to continue.

But even a less gifted runner can push his or her anaerobic threshold to the right of the scale: from 50 percent toward 85 percent. And speedwork is the way to do this.

FAST TWITCH VERSUS SLOW TWITCH

Not all of us are born physiologically equal, and it is true that some possess more natural speed than others. David L. Costill, PhD, popularized the theory of fast-twitch versus slow-twitch muscles. Everybody is blessed with both, but some have more of one than the other. Along with biomechanical differences, this is one reason why some people succeed as sprinters and others as distance runners.

Fast-twitch muscles fire quickly, of course, but they also quickly exhaust their supply of fuel in the form of glycogen. Fast-twitch muscles are geared for short bursts of energy. Think Olympic gold medalist Usain Bolt running the 100-meter dash. Slow-twitch muscles contract more slowly, but they maintain that contraction for a longer period of time. Think Olympian Paula Radcliffe running the marathon. Long-distance runners such as Radcliffe have more slow-twitch muscles that excel for activities that require continuous effort.

Along with these two basic types, scientists recognize a third type of muscle that fits somewhere in the middle: a fast-twitch muscle that can be trained for endurance, or a slow-twitch muscle that can be trained for speed. In an article for *Esquire* magazine on the subject, Kevin Shyne wrote, "Although it's long been believed that the ratio of fast- to slow-twitch fibers is genetically determined, a number of coaches and sports scientists have recently challenged that view. They hold that speed is much more learnable than previously believed and that anyone can substantially improve his ability to run fast through proper training."

Coach Glover adds, "Many runners, especially beginning racers, underestimate their abilities as athletes. Through speed training, they often discover that they are tougher than they had realized."

Apart from its physiological considerations, I look upon speedwork as a fine-tuning device, a means by which you become able to extract the maximum amount of energy from an already well-conditioned machine, the human body. Speedwork is a training method that may allow you, after many months or even years of long, steady running, to continue to progress after you seem to have reached a performance plateau.

At the top competitive levels, speed also is important for tactical reasons. Former University of Oregon coach Bill Dellinger says, "The distance runner who has the potential to sprint at the end of a race has a distinct advantage. He can relax and allow the other runners to do all the pacing, relying on his ability to accelerate at the finish. It's known as a kick.

"The problem," he adds, "is that distance runners spend hundreds of hours and thousands of miles training, yet neglect that one weapon—acceleration, or the ability to sprint—that all would love to have."

TYPES OF SPEEDWORK

There are various forms of speedwork. Some of them are quite difficult, some of them quite easy, some of them quite similar, some of them quite different. Different coaches have favored certain forms over others, based partly on their own intuitive perception of what works best for their runners. And a form of speedwork that works best for one runner may not necessarily work best for another.

Some forms of speedwork are best for improving strength; others, for improving endurance. Some help you with your form; others, with your concentration. Another important consideration is the confidence that comes from training hard in a measured environment. How you conduct your speed sessions may depend on your specific situation and surroundings. Your training plans will be dictated by whether you live near a track, a golf course, or a wooded area with trails, for example. Weather conditions may be a factor, as will be the length and importance of the race for which you're training.

In this chapter, I'll cover one type of speedwork, called repeats. In the chapters ahead, I'll also describe intervals, sprints, strides, surges, fartlek, and hill training—and how to successfully implement and use them in your training schedule.

Repeats

A repeat workout is one in which you run very fast, usually over a very short distance, and take a relatively long period of time to recover before repeating that distance again.

Running repeats was the first type of training I encountered when I went out for track as a youngster. It was a simple, basic method for working on your speed, one employed by sprinters as well as distance runners.

Repeat running, as taught by many track coaches, was a fairly unsophisticated form of training. It was easy for a coach to pull out a stopwatch and tell his runners to sprint a fast lap. After timing the runners, he could tell them to "walk it off" while he gave his attention to the high jumpers or shot-putters. Looking up 5 minutes later, he would see his runners standing around and send them sprinting around the track again.

At a luncheon in New York, Glenn Cunningham, America's greatest miler in the 1930s, described to me the training methods that had brought him close to 4 minutes for that distance. Cunningham ran little else but repeats, claiming he rarely ran more than a dozen miles a week. A typical Cunningham workout was to sprint 220 yards as fast as he could. After resting, he would sprint another 220, then go home. All of the milers from that era trained similarly.

I graduated from college in 1953 and, during graduate school, trained with the late coach Ted Haydon at the University of Chicago. Haydon patterned his training after that of Billy Hayes, the successful Indiana University coach whose runners included Don Lash and two time Olympian Fred Wilt. After a run of 3 miles on Mondays, we would do three or four 440-meter runs on Tuesdays, a couple of 880s on Wednesdays, five or six 220s on Thursdays, rest on Fridays, and race 2 miles on Saturdays, taking Sundays off. Although it was not identified as such, our training consisted mostly of repeats, because we paid little attention to what we did between fast runs. We recovered by jogging, walking, or sometimes, sitting down.

In 1956, I traveled to Berlin to participate as a member of a U.S. team in the Conseil Internationale du Sport Militaire (CISM) Championships, a track-and-field meet for athletes serving in the armed forces of various nations. On our team was Tom Courtney, a Fordham University graduate who would win the 800 meters at the Melbourne Olympic Games later that year, running 1:47.7. He also had won the National AAU 400 title that same year.

I would like to tell you that I trained with Courtney, but as someone with considerably less speed, I mostly watched as he ran through a series of 300-meter repeats. Even then, long, long before there was a *Runner's World* magazine, I was curious about training, the type of workouts that would allow me to run faster. Luckily, most other runners were happy to discuss and compare their training methods, even with arch rivals. Tom explained that he would begin the track season running 8 × 300; then as he got fitter and faster, he would actually cut the number, but run each repeat faster. At peak training, he would run 3 × 300 at full speed. (Full speed for Courtney was 45.0 for 400 meters, still fast more than a half century later.)

It seemed like a reasonable way to train, so eventually I copied Courtney's workout, modifying it to my own needs as a distance runner. I developed a pattern for repeat running, which I described as "three times something." Three became my magic number. I rarely did more, because too many repetitions converted a speed workout into an endurance workout. My body quickly told me that to do more than three, I would need to slow down. The purpose of the workout was to run near maximum speed. There was nothing scientific about my approach; it simply felt right.

ADD SPEEDWORK CAREFULLY

Bob Williams, a coach from Portland, Oregon, warns against adding speed training, or any different type of training, too quickly to your workout schedule. "Begin with one day of speedwork a week," advises Williams. "Allow at least six weeks to gradually adapt your body to this change of pace."

As an example, Williams suggests that a miler might begin with 4 × 400 meters and bit by bit build up to 8 × 400 meters. "Don't let the total mileage get too high," warns Williams.

A 5K or 10K runner might take a slightly different approach, using 800-meter repeats instead of 400-meter repeats. Marathoners might do 1-mile or even 2-mile repeats. Williams suggests that a 10K runner not do more than half the race distance at speed (thus 5K or a dozen 400 meters on the track as maximum).

"There's no perfect rule that suggests how fast you can progress, or how much speedwork you can tolerate in any one session or during a week," says Williams. "If you begin conservatively, there's less chance you will get hurt. Be particularly careful about mixing volume and intensity, a sure formula for disaster."

Typical workouts that I used were: 3 × 200, 3 × 300, and 3 × 400, or for variation, a 200, a 300, and a 400. I seldom went beyond one lap on a track in a single repeat, although years ago, one of my favorite workouts was to crowd 3 flat-out miles within the space of an hour. Were I to do that workout today, it would probably be over a measured road course. At peak training, I included one repeat workout in my schedule each week—but never exactly the same workout. For psychological reasons, I did not want to be able to look at this week's workout and realize that I ran one-tenth second slower than last week.

Owen Anderson, PhD, an exercise scientist and former columnist for *Runner's World*, recommends that each rest period be about five times as long as it takes you to run each fast repeat. This 1-to-5 ratio sounds about right to me. Usually, I would rest by walking the same distance that I had just run. After finishing a 300, I would turn and walk back to where I had started. If I felt I needed more recovery time after I got back to the starting line, I would take it. While coaching high school runners, I sometimes found that they liked to jog and walk back to the start, anxious to go again. I'd hold them to a 5-minute break to be certain they were well rested. I would watch them and talk to them, and if they looked like they needed more time, I would give them more time. I stressed to them, and I stress to you, that repeats should not be a punishing workout. You should finish a repeat workout refreshed and feeling positive about running hard with good form.

CONTROL INTENSITY FOR BEST RESULTS

One word of caution (I mentioned it before, but it's important enough to say again): Runners new to speedwork (including masters runners) should not begin by running repeats flat out. Build your speedwork the way you build your distance. Start easily and gradually increase the pace for the full length of the repeat. Over a period of weeks and months, improve your total time by gradually accelerating toward the end of each repeat. Try to maintain enough control so you can finish each repeat at a speed faster than you start.

In training runners in Dallas, Robert Vaughan, PhD, has them run 400s with the second 200 faster than the first. If you finish your repeats struggling and with your form deteriorating, you're running too far, too fast, or doing too many repeats. Pick a distance, speed, and number that you can run while maintaining good speed and form. If you allow your form to get sloppy from fatigue, you may find yourself plagued with sloppy form in races.

That's one reason I like 300 meters as a distance for repeats. It's longer than the sprint distances of 100 and 200 meters, so you don't (or shouldn't) run it full speed. And it's shorter than 400 meters, so you stop before lactic acid slows your pace and tightens your legs.

On most tracks, the start for the 300 meters is after the first turn, at the beginning of the back straightaway. That's also the start for the 1500 meters. I recommended that my track athletes begin relatively slowly in the first 100 meters down the back straightaway, build through the second 100 meters coming around the turn, and then kick the final 100 meters down the home straightaway. I ask them to visualize running the last 300 meters of their races. Repeats thus become an exercise to fine-tune a finishing kick. When the runners reach that point in a race, they can relate their kick to the repeats they run in practice.

At Indiana University, track coach Sam Bell used a similar philosophy, but he fine-tuned his runners using 150-meter sprints. Bell coached a series of fine milers on his teams, including a world championship silver medalist, Jim Spivey (a teammate of my son Kevin). Coach Bell felt that the last turn and final straightaway of a 1500 is where the race is won or lost. Regardless of the distance you choose for repeats, they should be done with control.

In an article translated from Russian and published in *Track Technique* magazine, former Russian coach A. Yakimov advises, "Repetition training is not a sprint nor a run at full strength. The athlete runs at a set and controlled pace, which depends on what distance and pace he is preparing himself for. This type of training is a method for developing speed and speed endurance, and can be considered as a method used to develop tempo and a sense of pace. Repetition training brings out a reaction from the body similar to that of a race. So this method finds its main use in the competitive season."

USE REST INTERVALS WISELY

"Some runners rest sitting down," Yakimov continues. "[With] this, they have noticed that the [runner's] heart rate drops to normal faster than when jogging. However, the recovery of the [runner's] heart rate is not the only important issue. It's possible that it's better to jog than to sit, especially after an intense run. Slow running offers the muscles a massaging effect, which helps clear waste products and increase the supply to the muscles of oxygen and sugar. In repetition work, the rest should consist of jogging followed by walking, and then sitting or lying down."

When doing repeat miles on the track while at the University of Chicago, I'd walk or jog over to the gymnasium and lie down on the wrestling mats during my 20-minute recovery period. This had the advantage of getting me out of the heat and the sun, since I usually did this workout in midsummer. Later as a masters runner, while running repeat 400s, I sometimes would continue around the track, walking 100 meters, jogging 200 meters down the back straightaway and around the turn, then walking 100 meters down the home straightaway before running hard again.

Why? Because it feels right. Every runner needs to determine the best form of rest for his or her particular needs. What's important is that you rest, but how you rest is up to you.

Yakimov notes that lengthening the rest intervals (within certain limits) and going faster on the runs increases the workout's effect on your speed. Conversely, shortening the rest periods and slowing the runs decreases the effect on your speed and increases the influence on your endurance.

The table on the following page shows the rest intervals recommended by Yakimov and can help you determine how long to rest during various forms of speed training. You also can use the table for interval training (see Chapter 13).

Had Yakimov included my favorite distance, 300 meters, in his table, his rest period would probably have come close to matching the 5-minute rest I suggest. When I ran 3 × 1 mile, my rest periods were close to the 20 minutes that Yakimov recommends for runners doing 2000-meter repeats, which are a quarter-mile longer. What many coaches determine scientifically, runners learn intuitively. Actually, the best coaches simply watch the workouts done by intuitive runners, learn from them, and systemize their training for the benefit of other runners.

Rest Periods

DISTANCE OF FAST RUN (METERS)	LENGTH OF REST (MINUTES)		
	EASY PACE	HARD PACE	FLAT-OUT PACE
100	Up to 0:30	Up to 0:30	Up to 3:00
200	1:00	2:00	4:00
400	1:30	3:00	7:00
800	2:30	5:00	9:00
1000	3:00	6:00	12:00
1200	4:00	7:00	15:00
2000	5:00	8:00	20:00

SHARPEN YOUR RUNNING ECONOMY

Repeats also promote running economy. Writing in *Runner's World* magazine, Dr. Anderson describes research by a team of exercise scientists from Arizona State University that followed miler Steve Scott's training over a period of 9 months.

Scott improved his running economy by 5 percent, but, Dr. Anderson suggests, only after he added fast 200- to 600-meter runs to his training program. After improving his economy, Scott set two United States records: 3:31.96 for the 1500 meters and 3:49.68 for the mile.

"The key to improving economy is to run fast while you're feeling strong and relaxed, not when you're tired and struggling and your running style is unnatural and fatigued," Dr. Anderson advises.

CHAPTER THIRTEEN

THE MAGIC WORKOUT
Interval training can improve your speed

On a warm evening in autumn my grandson, Kyle Higdon, heads to the track. It is an odd track, distanced 444 yards instead of the more familiar 440 yards, or 400 meters. Three unmarked lanes. Uphills and downhills. What Kyle describes as "squiggly/sharp turns." He explains: "We need to contest with walkers and joggers for the inside lane, but they learn quickly to get out of the way of faster runners coming up from behind."

Kyle is among the third generation of Higdon runners, which started with me. His father Kevin ran for Indiana University and qualified for the 1984 Olympic Trial marathon with a time of 2:18:50. Kyle ran cross-country and track for Michigan City High School and the University of Notre Dame before moving to Austin. Various uncles and aunts and siblings and cousins and friends and neighbors and girlfriends run. But on this evening, Kyle's mission at the track was not to train himself for some future race, but to train others.

In his spare time, Kyle serves as a volunteer coach for the Texas Running Club (TRC), which is affiliated with the University of Texas. In recent years, many colleges have downgraded their varsity programs, abandoning the inclusive anybody-can-run approach. Athletic directors often force coaches to limit their programs to a dozen or more extremely talented scholarship runners, leaving moderately talented runners out. Fortunately, the same schools have begun to promote club teams that are open to anyone who wants to participate. Some even participate in national club championships.

The Texas Running Club fulfills this need in Austin. In the several years that Kyle has served as volunteer coach, he brought TRC from last place in the Intramural Track Meet to first place. The distance runners he coached dominated the meet, plus he got some valuable team points from several of the sprinters.

For this evening, Kyle chooses a familiar workout for runners who are bent on fast running: interval training. At the track, and after warming up a group of nearly four dozen runners with jogging, stretching, and leg drills, Kyle divides everybody into three groups based on ability. The basic workout for a 5K/10K group and a marathon group is two sets of 4 × 400 meters, 200 meters between each 400 rep, 3 minutes between the sets. Sprinters do more of a speed-based workout.

In a similar workout a few weeks before, several runners had gone out faster than planned for the early reps, then struggled completing the workout. For this evening, Kyle stresses a slower start. This provides more consistent times throughout the workout, both for the reps and the intervals between the reps. In an e-mail to me, my grandson explained: "Everyone was pretty fatigued at the end, because it was uncharacteristically hot, but they recovered rapidly while stretching afterward and during a cooldown run, between a half and full mile barefoot on the infield."

Not only in Austin, but in many areas, from Eugene to Boulder to Albuquerque to Jacksonville to Chicago, runners look to the track—and interval training done on the track—as a major method for improving performance. Perhaps no other workout promises better benefits than interval training.

> *No other workout promises better benefits than interval training.*

WHAT IS INTERVAL TRAINING?

"Contrary to popular belief," says Bill Dellinger, the legendary former coach at the University of Oregon, "interval training isn't superfast, all-out running as much as it is controlled running." Control, of course, is important in

REPEAT TRAINING VERSUS INTERVAL TRAINING

How does repeat training differ from interval training? Runners sometimes get these two important forms of speed training confused. Little wonder, because the difference between them is relatively small, and the overlap is great.

First, a couple of definitions. A "repeat" (or "rep") is the fast portion of the workout. An "interval" is what goes on between repeats.

In interval training, the runner runs his or her reps fast, but the runner runs faster in repeat training. In interval training, the runner usually runs more reps, say a dozen, compared with repeat training where the runner runs fewer repeats, say three. In interval training, the runner takes less rest between reps than in repeat training, where the runner takes more rest.

Still confused? Let's compare a repeat workout with an interval workout. First, a typical workout of repeats for a fast runner:

3 × 400 meters in 60 seconds, 5-minute rest between.

And here is a typical interval workout for that same runner:

12 × 400 meters in 70 seconds, 2-minute rest between.

The difference between the two workouts seems insignificant, but coaches (and their runners) use repeat workouts to improve speed—pure speed. And while interval workouts also will improve speed, the focus tilts more to building endurance—or as Russell H. Pate, PhD, of the University of South Carolina might say, speed endurance.

Is it possible to fill the gap between the two types of speed workouts? Yes, it is. If you take that first 3 × 400 workout and over a period of several weeks bump the number to 4 × 400, then up to 5 × 400 and to 6 × 400 and beyond, it begins to look like the second interval workout. This is particularly true since you probably will need to slow down from 60 to 61 to 62 seconds and beyond to continue the workout. Another compounding variable would be how much you rest between each repeat. (See Gerschler and Dr. Reindell's five variables on page 127.)

The difference between these two forms of speed training is less than it might seem. Both workouts effectively improve speed and both workouts should be included in any balanced training program.

any intelligent training program. The subtle difference between running repeats (page 113) and doing interval training—other than the fact that you usually include more repetitions in the latter—is that you *control* the rest interval between the fast runs as well as the speed and distance you are running.

That's an important point. The key word is *between*. Many runners mistakenly refer to intervals as the fast part of the speedwork. ("I ran my intervals in 70 seconds a lap.") Not so. Check any dictionary. The term *interval* is defined as an intervening period of time, a period of temporary cessation, a pause.

Remember that. The interval is the rest that happens between the fast running. The fast run is more properly referred to as the repetition (although this term could be confused with repeats). Many coaches call the fast segments reps.

> *"Interval training isn't superfast, all-out running as much as it is controlled running."*

But what's more important than what you call them is why you do them and how you do them.

THE VALUE OF INTERVAL TRAINING

Certainly, the value of interval training has been recognized for more than half a century, dating back to the late 1930s when the German coach Waldemar Gerschler asked his top athlete Rudolf Harbig to train by running alternate fast and slow laps. In 1939, Harbig ran a world record 1:46.6 for 800 meters, a mark that remained on the books for nearly two decades.

Tom Ecker, an expert on coaching techniques from Iowa, once described interval training as "the most effective single training system ever devised."

David L. Costill, PhD, claims that a runner shifting to interval training often can improve speed after only a single session.

Bill Dellinger states, "Interval training—if it's done properly—develops speed in a runner more quickly than any other form of training."

The magic workout? The title for this chapter is aptly chosen. If I had to name one single type of training capable of converting a plodder into a runner, this would be it. Remember what I wrote in in previous chapters about my clubmate Joanne Kittel, the novice who became a gazelle after using quarter-mile marks for speed workouts? Well those speed workouts were in fact a form of interval training. When carefully structured into a well-designed workout regimen, interval training may not necessarily turn you into an Olympian, but it can make you a faster runner.

An article by Brian Mitchell in *Athletics Weekly* magazine presents the case for interval training. "In this type of (training), the runner gets the best of two worlds because he keeps moving throughout and is able regularly to raise the pace above what would be done in a steady run, and thereby also extend the range of body movement, with all that implies for muscles and nerves. The session is under as much control as you want. It is systematic and definite, and it is tailored for each individual, so long as he does not allow himself to be overrun by a group of fellow athletes and forced to go their pace rather than his own."

The interval is the rest that happens between the fast running.

Mitchell adds, "Interval training can also be intelligently progressive, month by month, season by season, accessible and adjustable."

If proof were needed of the effectiveness of interval training, James Stray-Gundersen, MD, provided it during a study he did in collaboration with Peter Snell, PhD, at the University of Texas in Dallas. The two researchers asked 10 experienced runners, whose 10K times averaged between 34 and 42 minutes (fast, but not superfast), to train for 6 weeks at 50 miles a week, building a base. Dr. Stray-Gundersen and Dr. Snell divided the runners: One group did a form of lactate threshold training (fast repeats, more than ample rest between). The other group did interval work (400s in 75 to 85 seconds, 200s in 33 to 38 seconds).

At the end of 10 weeks of training, the researchers tested both groups by having them race at 800- and 10,000-meter distances. Analysis showed that the interval-trained group improved their 800 times by 11.2 seconds and their 10,000 times by more than 2 minutes. The lactate threshold training group demonstrated lesser improvements: 6.6 seconds in the 800 and just over 1 minute in the 10,000. Improvements in VO_2 max showed a similar division: 12 percent in the interval group, 4 percent in the lactate threshold group.

The study featured a small sampling, so keep that in mind when considering the findings. Knowing how scientists behave, and having attended numerous American College of Sports Medicine meetings, I can almost visualize one or more doubters muttering the words "statistically insignificant" under their breath. But I know Dr. Stray-Gundersen and Dr. Snell well, and I feel they are onto something when they identify interval training as a top ranking form of speedwork.

Dr. Stray-Gundersen and Dr. Snell worked with well-conditioned runners, but they are not the only researchers to have studied the subject of intervals. At the University of Miami, Arlette C. Perry, PhD, tested 66 college-age women in an aerobic dance class, training two groups 3 days a week for 35 minutes a day at 75 to 85 percent of their MHR. The control group did aerobics for 35 minutes nonstop. The interval group alternated 3 to 5 minutes of aerobics with brisk walking, which stretched the workout past 35 minutes.

Before telling you the results, let me impress on you that the form of training used by Dr. Perry closely resembles the run/walk approach I suggested for beginning runners earlier in this book. (See Chapter 3.)

After 12 weeks, the control group had improved cardiovascular endurance by 8 percent; the interval group had improved by 18 percent. Other studies at the University of Massachusetts and Arizona State University showed similar benefits for interval training.

But is this a training method that can benefit every runner? What about someone whose only goal, admirably, is to nibble a few seconds off her 5K time, not win an Olympic medal? Let's discuss this magic training method in greater detail.

MEET WALDERMAR GERSCHLER

German coach Waldermar Gerschler, who trained Rudolf Harbig to his 800 world record, is credited with the development of interval training as an important means of improving speed and endurance. Gerschler was not the first coach to ask his athletes to alternate fast and slow running. Earlier, the Finnish coach Lauri Pikhala had developed a system of "terrace training," which consisted of repeated speed runs with slower running between.

Czechoslovakia's Emil Zatopek also employed this pattern in his training, running as much as 60 × 400 meters, although slower than race pace. After Zatopek's three victories at the 1952 Olympics in Helsinki (5000, 10,000, marathon), coaches and athletes began to examine his training methods. They realized the biggest advantage of fast/slow training: Runners could work at race paces and with race intensities by utilizing recovery segments midworkout.

Gerschler's contribution was to systemize interval training, which he did in collaboration with Hans Reindell, MD, a cardiologist. Reportedly, Gerschler and Dr. Reindell studied more than 3,000 individuals. According to an article by Paul A. Smith in *Athletics Journal,* the German coach and physician together pinpointed when the greatest stimulus for heart development occurs—during the first 10 seconds of the recovery interval. "The run provides the stress, while the interval allows for the development response," Smith explained. "Because Gerschler and Dr. Reindell realized during their research that the rest period was the key to development, they named this exercise interval training." And it became a successful formula for improving speed and endurance that could be applied to almost any workout at any level.

In describing interval training, Gerschler and Dr. Reindell identified the following variables. (I reference the heartrate numbers used in their study, rather than the percentages.)

1. **Distance.** How far you run during each repetition. Gerschler and Dr. Reindell determined that the time for each run should not exceed 90 seconds. (This suggested a distance no longer than 600 meters, although 400 meters, one lap around the track, became the distance most favored by runners for interval workouts.) The intensity should be sufficient to produce a heart rate of 170 to 180 beats per minute, which they measured during the first 10 seconds of the recovery period. This was 85 to 90 percent of the MHR for the young athletes measured.

2. **Interval.** How long you rest during each interval. They also deduced that the interval should not exceed 90 seconds. They noted that it took

only 30 seconds into the interval for the pulse to drop to approximately 130 beats per minute (the equivalent of 65 to 70 percent of their MHRs). If the pulse failed to fall below 140, they slowed the pace or shortened the distance. If the pulse remained elevated, they stopped the workout.

3. **Repetitions.** How many times you run the distance. (Or, in coaching jargon, how many reps.)

4. **Pace.** How fast you run the specified distance.

5. **Rest.** What you do during the interval.

Let me offer you an example based on my own training past. While researching the first edition of this book, I visited the National Institute for Fitness and Sport in Indianapolis to interview exercise physiologist Dean Brittenham. It was December, and I arrived early to use the institute's indoor track: 200 meters, approximately eight laps to the mile. The institute is located a short distance from the Indiana University–Purdue University in Indianapolis (IUPUI) outdoor track, which has been used for many national championships and Olympic Trials.

For various reasons, I decided that morning to run 300-meter repetitions, a lap and a half on the track. Thus, that became my distance, the first variable. The distance usually remains constant during any single workout, but may vary from one workout to the next. "The important thing," says Tom Ecker, "is that the distance is shorter than the athlete's race distance, usually in multiples of 100."

At the institute, fast runners are asked to use the outside lanes, leaving the inside lanes for walkers and joggers. I chose lane 5, which meant that after finishing each 300, I would need to continue around the track approximately another 140 meters to get back to the starting line. This became my interval, the second variable.

Not knowing how I would feel, since this was my first run on the institute's track, I simply ran until I felt I had a good workout. I stopped after 11 repetitions, the third variable. "The exact number of runs is not important," says Ecker. "The important thing is that they have been run to their absolute limit." Ecker considers this the biggest guessing game the coach (or athlete) has to play. "If too low (the number of reps) reduces the effectiveness of the workout," he says. "If too high, the runner crashes."

My time for each 300 was around 61 or 62 seconds—although borrowing a tip from coach Dellinger, I ran two of my reps (the 6th and the 11th) faster, 58 and 56 seconds. The pace I ran was the fourth variable. "The speed of each repeat run," suggests Ecker, "is determined by the runner's projected race pace."

Between reps, I jogged at a moderate speed, covering the 140-meter interval distance in 60 to 65 seconds. That converts to approximately 12-minute miles, 5 mph. When I was a younger and faster runner, I usually ran my intervals at a pace of 8:00 per mile, jogging 400 meters in 2:00, which I shamefacedly now confess put me outside Gerschler's 90-second barrier for rest. But then I was only an ordinary athlete whose training had not yet been analyzed by scientists.

The rest between bouts of running fast was the fifth and final variable. "For interval training to be a truly effective system for conditioning the runner's cardiorespiratory system," says Ecker, "the heart rate must be alternately increased during the runs and decreased to a level of semirecovery between runs."

This resulted in a rather neat workout package: 1 minute of hard running followed by 1 minute of easy running, repeated 11 times. A workout that, not counting warm-up and cool-down time, lasted 22 minutes. A very efficient package. My heart rate on the fast runs rose to above 90 percent of my MHR; during the intervals, it dropped to 70 percent of my MHR. (Keep in mind that my maximum heart rate back then was a very low and well-trained 150 or slightly higher.)

In shortened form, the workout could be described as: 11 × 300 (61.1 seconds average), 140 rest between (65.1 seconds average). That sounds scientific, but actually, I just showed up at the track and did what my body told me was a reasonable workout for my level of training and my feelings of energy on that particular morning. I might add that I finished the workout comfortably, feeling that I put in some hard work that felt good, whether or not it would help me in my next race. Most runners who use interval training realize that there is an exhilaration that these workouts provide, what might be called higher than the usual runner's high.

That single well-measured workout would provide a database for future workouts. One week later, I was in New York City on business and worked out one morning on the cinder path (approximately 2,000 meters around) that circles the reservoir in Central Park. I set my watch to beep every 60 seconds to remind me to alternate running fast and slow. I ran 11 fast sprints in this manner, jogging between. My measured heart rates were

CONTROLLED CHAOS

In coaching the Texas Running Club, my grandson Kyle used one workout that I found fascinating. He would begin by dividing runners into relay teams, with each team having three members. The first runner, usually a marathon runner, ran 600 meters, then hand-tapped a second runner, usually a middle-distance runner, who would run 400 meters, then hand-tap a third runner, usually a sprinter, who would run 200 meters, then hand-tap to the first runner, who would begin his second repetition. Each individual on the team would run a total of 6 reps, thus: 6 × 600; 6 × 400; or 6 × 200.

Most interesting, the marathon runners ran the farthest distances and had the shortest rest. Because of this, they also ran the slowest pace. At the other end, the sprinters ran the shortest distances and had the most rest. Because of this, they also ran the fastest pace. The middle-distance runners fit between. Not the type of workout that an individual runner might do, but for a group of 30 to 40 runners, it was perfect. Most important: relay running is fun. I liked the fact that it provided controlled chaos.

Kyle claimed this to be a workout of repeats, not interval training. He is probably correct, although you might say that the workout occupied a position somewhere in the middle. But does it matter what we call a workout as long as it is enjoyable and gets you in shape? We need all the tools in our toolboxes that are available to us.

slightly lower than in Indianapolis, possibly because chilly weather prevented me from going full tilt. Otherwise, this New York workout was a carbon copy of the workout in Indianapolis. While interval training most often is done on the track, it need not always be.

WHY DO INTERVAL TRAINING?

Interval running, even at relatively slow speeds, is more demanding than ordinary running. It is a high-stress workout. It also can be more time consuming. You may need to travel to a track, or somewhere flat and marked, to do it. You need to spend more time warming up and cooling down and stretching so that you can run fast without getting injured. So why train that hard when jogging in the park or nonstop around the New York reservoir is more fun and less stressful?

The main reason for interval training, of course, is improvement. A secondary reason might be pleasure. Yes, what seems painful can also be fun. Although some may consider interval training painful, it actually can be a rather benign way to train at race pace. Certainly, running 400 meters at your best pace for 10,000 meters, then slowing down to rest before taking on another 400, is easier than running 25 laps at your best possible pace. Practically all research done on distance runners suggests that they improve when they add intensity to their programs.

The other side of that coin, of course, is a study of walkers and joggers executed by the late Michael L. Pollock, PhD, who was director of the University of Florida's Center for Exercise Science. Dr. Pollock's study showed that intensity is exactly what scares beginners away. Dr. Pollock also believed that it subjects them to higher injury risk, although I'm not entirely sure I agree. At the American College of Sports Medicine meeting one year, I had a conversation with a pair of New Zealand scientists who claimed interval-trained runners were less prone to injury, according to a study they had conducted. Nevertheless, when you mention intensity or interval training to the people who run with no other goal other than a new T-shirt in 5K races, their attention sometimes drops. They don't want to go fast or do speedwork; they just want to get in their daily 5 miles and burn a few calories to feel good and look good.

If that is your approach, don't change. Yet beyond a desire to improve race times, those who embrace intensity comprehend that there is a mystical aspect to interval training. It can be exhilarating—it can improve your concentration and refine your technique and form. Interval training done in the company of like-minded fellow runners results in a shared experience, even if you're too stressed during or afterward to talk. Running with the Texas Running Club, simply stated, is fun! Ask my grandson Kyle. Runners like each other's company. They can talk about the previous weekend's 5K race. Medals in their closet. Boyfriends. Girlfriends. Food trucks to visit. Food trucks to avoid. Being able to see improvement from week to week—both in yourself and in others—also offers a form of motivation and a topic for conversation.

MORE ART THAN SCIENCE

How fast should you run in interval training? That's a tricky question, despite all the expert advice and the charts published in running magazines that seem to offer exact answers. An experienced coach, observing you in training over a period of 6 months or more, might be able to tell you how fast to run—or he might not. Coaching remains somewhat of a guessing game; it's more art than science. People differ in their abilities, and they also differ in their ability to train hard on the track. Someone new to interval training certainly would find it more stressful than an old warhorse like myself. And not every day is equal to every other day. Outdoors, weather can affect workouts. It could be hot or humid or cold or windy. You might arrive at the track fatigued from a hard day of work or too little sleep the night before because one of your kids was sick. What you ran the day before, whether hard or easy, also can affect your training. As a result, it's sometimes difficult to compare one week's workout with the next—although over a period of time, a pattern usually does emerge.

People differ in their abilities, and they also differ in their ability to train hard on the track.

Jim Huff, a coach with the Motor City Striders in Detroit, once warned against setting too-precise goals for interval workouts. "Runners get frustrated if you say run a certain speed and they can't accomplish that, so any time set has to be realistic," he explains. "You can't just read what other people do and try to copy their workouts."

Owen Anderson, PhD, an exercise scientist and former columnist for *Runner's World*, suggests in his publication *Running Research News* that interval training be carried out at an intensity of 90 to 100 percent of your MHR—about the same intensity as a 10K race. I liked Owen's percentage-based approach better than I do that of scientists who quote heartbeats. Thus, a good starting point for most people beginning interval training is to train at a slightly faster pace than you run in a 10K race, or at about the same pace you might run a 5K. Some coaches also suggest that if your racing goal is a 5K, then you should train at your speed for the mile or 1500 meters. Milers should train at half-mile pace, and so forth.

Because runners vary so greatly in ability, I usually use race pace (pace for a specific race distance) to define how fast to run in any interval workout. Thus an athlete capable of competing in the Olympic arena might run 400-meter reps in close to 60 seconds, while other runners might run 2 minutes or 3 minutes or more for their fast 400s.

Dr. Snell advises against running interval 400s at faster than race pace. During my competitive years, I used to violate that rule frequently, but I am convinced now that Dr. Snell got it right. "It is tempting to run fast during your workouts," he says, "but remember that you're not going to be able to run that fast in a race. If you run too fast during workouts, you'll get too fatigued to do good training, and you'll also get out of your race rhythm. Too much speed is more damaging than too much distance."

Training at race pace does have another important advantage. You develop pace judgment. During the phase of my running career when I ran a lot of intervals, I could almost tell how fast I had run each 400-meter lap without even looking at my watch or waiting for the coach beside the track to call my time. I had a well-developed internal clock, similar to that possessed by people who wake up two minutes before the alarm goes off.

On occasion, I've participated in "prediction miles," where the winner is not the fastest runner but rather the one able to predict his or her time.

The enviable purpose, of course, is to allow less experienced runners to win a few awards in an event where speed is not a factor. Inevitably, the fastest runners still win, because they are most likely to have honed their pace judgment through interval training. In one prediction mile, I embarrassed myself and got all the other contestants upset by selecting a time somewhere around 9 minutes, finishing well behind almost everybody who entered, yet still winning because I nailed my time within a few seconds. One year, I led a pacing team for *Runner's World* magazine at the Walt Disney World Marathon and hit five of my mile splits within 1 second of perfect while bringing a group of several hundred runners home almost exactly on time.

My ability to tell you exactly the pace I'm running has recently faded somewhat because I am less competition-oriented than I was years before. But I still possess a well-developed ability to sense pace changes of even a few seconds per mile by others running around me in races. This is an important skill because running at a consistent speed is one way to conserve energy.

> *"Too much speed is more damaging than too much distance."*

SETTING REALISTIC GOALS

When he coached at the University of Oregon, Bill Dellinger utilized a system of interval training that he borrowed from his predecessor, Bill Bowerman. The system revolved around "date pace" and "goal pace." Date pace is the pace at which you can currently run your race distance. Goal pace is the pace at which you hope to run that distance toward the end of the season—that is, in the important meets. For top University of Oregon runners, that meet was the NCAA championships. My most important race of the year often was the World Masters Athletics Championships (for over-40 runners), where I often ran the 5000 meters, or sometimes the 3000-meter or 2000-meter steeplechase. To fine-tune my speed for those distances, I would also do several 1500-meter races leading up to that meet. So in doing interval training, I needed to work at paces I would be running in races that ranged between 1500 and 5000 meters.

When I threw those two fast 300s into the middle of my workout in Indianapolis, I actually was following a variation of the University of Oregon interval system. I was running the reps at a pace near what I felt I could accomplish at that time. A 300-meter pace of 61.1 maintained for 1500 meters would give me a final time of 5:05.6 for that distance (date pace). However, if I could maintain the 58.7 I ran in my sixth quarter, or the 56.2 I ran in my final quarter, I could run 4:53.5 or 4:41.0, respectively (goal pace).

I was far from being in peak shape during that midwinter workout in Indianapolis, but I had run 4:53.3 the previous August at the Masters Track and Field Championships in the same city. At the same meet in San Diego the year before, I had run 4:45.9, placing third, even though the 1500, or metric mile, was far from being my best event. For the coming year, a world championship year, I was setting my pace higher, so that day's training in Indianapolis seemed quite compatible with my plan. And, indeed, later that summer I placed first in the steeplechase at the World Masters Championships in Turku, Finland. All of that hard work on the Indianapolis track and on other tracks leading up to that meet did pay off.

I should repeat that I did not set out that morning in Indianapolis to run date pace and goal pace. I simply got out on the track and ran, allowing my body—essentially, how I was feeling—to set the effort of the workout. I was able to do that because of the experience I gained from decades of interval training.

Less experienced runners need to set their date and race paces for interval workouts more carefully. Bowerman believed that runners should feel exhilarated, not exhausted, at the end of a workout. "Too many individuals," he said, "simply run themselves into the ground and aren't fresh enough to race properly." He felt that if runners overwork, they become less excited about racing.

That's assuming that racing is the most important reason that you run. For the college coach, the race—whether during cross-country season or part of a track meet—certainly is the raison d'être of running. This was particularly true for Bowerman in 1972, the year he served as head track-and-field coach for the US Olympic team. If your end goal is to develop

Olympic champions, then certainly interval training provides a very effective means to that end.

But 1972 was the year that Frank Shorter won the Olympic Marathon in Munich. Shorter's victory was not the only reason for the running boom that followed soon after, but coincidentally, it did broaden the sport of running to a much wider field of participants with diverse goals. Not every runner has Shorter's talent, or even a fraction of that talent. Not every runner is training for an Olympic medal. Life for most runners today is more than an endless quest for medals or race T-shirts. Most of today's runners don't even race, and when they do, they run races more for social reasons than for success. We've redefined our goals since the time that Bowerman was coaching at

LEARNING TO LOVE SPEED

Does speed training work? Yes, according runners who have embraced this form of training and benefited from it.

"Speed work will make you or break you," admits Lionel Burnett, 55, an information technology manager and Road Runners Club of America certified coach from Fort Smith, Arkansas. He advises: "Be sure your form is good, and you will reap the rewards. However, speed work with bad form will leave you on the sideline waiting for your body to heal. Yes, I am speaking from experience on both counts."

Erin Edwards, from Duvail, Washington, admits to having a love/hate relationship with speedwork, saying: "I appreciate that speed training is different enough so that it forces me to think the entire time. I can't zone out. I need to be completely present. Not so on my weekend long runs."

In training for her first marathon, Adriana M. Treviño, from San Antonio, Texas, decided to train with a well-respected coach, Edgar Gonzalez of We Run San Antonio. She says, "I did my first speed workout last week at track practice and to my surprise I ran my fastest mile ever. I never knew I could run that fast. I'm looking forward to my next workouts on the track."

Oregon, so that the means are often more important than the end. The workout is more important than the race.

Coincidentally, Bowerman was one of the early pioneers in the fitness movement, teaching jogging to Eugene housewives as an aside to training elite athletes.

Perhaps I reflect my own philosophy, because I always have found myself able to secure as much masochistic enjoyment from a single well-crafted workout—a hard run in the park, a set of quarters strung together on the track—as from winning my age-group in a megarace. I still measure myself in megaraces, but hard running carries its own rewards. Interval training, because of the way it can be measured in bits and pieces, can provide a form

Denise Feinen, from Forestville, New York, used a unique approach while doing speed workouts on a treadmill. "I post a tic-tac-toe sheet on the treadmill and fill in the squares with a smiley face for each 400 completed. I used a novice marathon schedule with no speed workouts for my first marathon, then afterward used speedwork to get me back to my usual cadence and rhythm."

Hope Kirsch, from Casco, Michigan, describes using "a speedwork buddy" for her faster workouts: "It sometimes helps to race others of near ability. However, speedwork on my own has been very productive and I love it either way."

"Definitely not my favorite, and I'm not that fast," says Nancy Lehr, from Lawton, Oklahoma. That seems like a backhanded endorsement, but she adds, "I try to get some kind of speed workout in at least every other week. Realizing you can push yourself a little harder is a big confidence booster."

Larissa Martin Ralph, from Seattle, Washington, admits getting a "massive runner's high" from sprinting up hills, even though she does not always enjoy it. "Those sprints may be a killer, but I am in total bliss afterwards, knowing that they will help me reach my race goals."

of satisfaction akin to racing. Yes, those electronic devices that measure our pace and heart rate can both motivate and challenge us. That is not to say that dedicated coaches are wrong for their emphasis on racing as the end product. There is room within running for many philosophies. But you can enjoy running fast in workouts without necessarily pointing toward an upcoming race.

Nevertheless, there is nothing like competition to provide a level of motivation not experienced in practice. In describing a downhill ski race on television, Currie Chapman, retired coach of the Canadian National Women's Alpine Ski Team, suggested that the viewer should think of a string tied at the starting line and leading through the gates to the finish line. "In training," Chapman said, "there's slack in the string. Race day, adrenalin pulls the string tighter."

REACHING YOUR PEAK

Races provide a goal that can be approached with logical and systematic training. Interval training, of course, lends itself extremely well to progressive programs, ones in which you begin at a relatively low level of fitness and train progressively harder to improve performance. You go from weakness to strength via the overload principle. This can be accomplished in several ways.

In *Athletics Journal*, Donald E. Boggis Jr., a high school coach from Hollis, New Hampshire, discussed manipulation of the five variables in progressively overloading (and strengthening) the system. Boggis cited variables slightly different from those mentioned by coach Gerschler and others, but the effect is the same. As your training program progresses, suggests Boggis, you can increase the number of repetitions, or you can increase the speed you run them. You can decrease the amount of rest you take during the interval by jogging less, or you can increase the distance of the repetitions, maintaining the same pace. A wide variety of combinations present themselves.

Yet blind application of any number-based system can cause problems.

Fatigue, poor diet, and lack of sleep all can affect the intensity of your training. An additional variable—one not mentioned in most coaching articles—is weather. Cold, heat, wind, and rain can affect how fast or how far you run during any given workout.

Nevertheless, the advantage of training using an overload program is that it does provide a strong psychological carrot as you peak for a specific race. It's like runners in training for a marathon, who progressively increase the length of their weekend runs over a period of 18 weeks (if they use one of my schedules that utilizes that time period) to where they finally can cover 20 miles comfortably 3 weeks before they race 26. It's like the countdown before the launch of a space shuttle. After the long runs to develop endurance, after the fast runs to develop strength, you use a shot of speed training featuring intervals to fine-tune your speed. Because it lends itself to progressive manipulation (as suggested by Boggis), interval training offers an effective way of peaking.

Maintaining that peak is another matter. In discussing the benefits of interval training, Gerschler and Dr. Reindell commented, "Interval training saves time, is a good stimulant, but its disadvantage is that the achieved condition is not maintained for a long period."

Magic workout, you be the judge—but if you expect to run fast, you probably need to include some form of interval workouts in your regular training regimen.

FINDING MY WAY IN GERMANY

I first discovered the advantages of interval training while living in Germany in the mid-1950s. Gerschler was still training runners in that country at that time, but our paths never crossed. I knew him only by reputation.

I was a member of the United States Army, stationed in Germany from May 1955 to November 1956. I ran every day, not always with the Army's permission. While a member of the 63rd Tank Battalion in Kitzingen, I sometimes would crawl under a barbed-wire fence at the end of the day to run in a nearby forest. Later, while working as an ordinance draftsman at

Seventh Army Headquarters in Vaihingen, outside Stuttgart, I would appear at the camp exit at 9:00 p.m. dressed in my running gear. The guards at the gate probably thought I was crazy, but they waved me through when I showed them my pass. I remember those runs through what was truly the *Schwarzwald* (in English, the Black Forest) as among the most enjoyable workouts of my career. Spongy forest trails beneath my feet. Fir trees, which somehow I avoided bumping into, in a moonlight that made it magical.

On other occasions, usually on weekends, I would drive into town to train on the track of the VfB Stuttgart, a local sports club. Accompanying me was another soldier stationed at the post, Dean Thackwray, who made the 1956 US Olympic team in the marathon. Our frequent training partner was Stefan Lupfert, who won several German indoor championships at 3000 meters and also competed as a member of the national team in the 3000-meter steeplechase.

Dissatisfied with my previous training methods, I already had begun to increase the number of repetitions. But while training with Lupfert, I saw how he ran somewhat slower reps but jogged much faster between those reps, typically at about an 8-minute mile pace. A standard workout for our trio became 12 × 400, with a 400 jog between. The fast 400s were done in around 65 or 70 seconds, the slow 400 intervals in 2 minutes.

Also in Germany at that time was Frank McBride, whom I had run against in college when he competed for South Dakota State University in Brookings. McBride placed seventh in the 1500 meters at the 1952 US Olympic Trials, and he later achieved success as a masters runner. But at this period in his life, McBride was serving as a coach for Army runners stationed in Germany, first as an officer, later as a Department of the Army civilian. McBride was familiar with the theories of Gerschler and Dr. Reindell, and he encouraged me to use interval training. I found it to be a worthwhile program that cut more than a minute off my time for 5000 meters and several minutes off my time for 10,000 meters.

In all honesty, a major reason for my improvement was that in the previous year or two, I also had doubled the volume of my training to 100 miles a week. It sometimes is difficult to measure exactly why you improve. But certainly, all those nighttime runs in the *Schwarzwald* were having an effect. (That underlines the importance of building a good training base before beginning speedwork.) Nevertheless, interval training definitely was the key to my success. It was my magic workout.

GAINING AN EDGE WITH SLOW QUARTERS

Later, after my discharge from the Army, I returned home and began training at Stagg Field, the University of Chicago's track. It was also used by non-students, such as members of coach Ted Haydon's University of Chicago Track Club (UCTC).

Most runners training at the track—varsity and track club members—were more familiar with fast repeats. Like most American coaches, Haydon trained his runners in this manner: You ran a hard quarter around the track while the coach timed you. You then slowly walked or jogged once more around the track and waited until you caught his eye, so he could time you again for another hard quarter.

Interval training had only begun to penetrate the consciousness of the American distance runner. Other runners who decided to run quarters with me would sometimes become edgy about my seemingly slow pace and sprint ahead. By the end of the workout, they struggled to keep up—if they lasted to the end. They had not anticipated the stress imposed by the interval aspect of the workout. What tripped them up was not the fast reps, but the relatively fast interval jogging laps between the reps. (Thank you, Stefan Lupfert.) Sooner or later, the others became accustomed to this style of training—or found different training partners.

One Chicago runner who shared my enthusiasm for interval training was Gar Williams, who also had recently returned from service in Germany. Haydon used to chuckle at Williams for constantly running all those slow quarters.

Another UCTC member had placed high in the NCAA championships several years earlier. He trained in the old style, mostly fast repeats. I told Haydon that Williams would probably defeat the other runner later that season when we ran at the National AAU Track and Field Championships.

Haydon refused to believe me. Sure enough, Williams did what I had predicted. Eventually, Haydon and other American coaches came to appreciate the value of slow quarters. (Williams later won a National AAU marathon title and served a term as president of the Road Runners Club of America.)

The advantage of interval training—and one reason for its appeal to track coaches—is that it allows total control over the workout. It is very systematic, very precise. It is also a good means of charting your progress from week to week. If you record workouts in an app like Strava, Nike Plus, or Garmin, you can see that this week you ran your quarters in, say, an average of 75.3 seconds, compared with 76.1 last week, or 85.7 a couple of months ago. However, don't discount the value of such record-keeping by hand, or what might be called the Refrigerator Approach, since many runners check workouts off calendar schedules that are attached to their refrigerators with magnets. Regardless, one reason you succeed with your running is confidence: a belief in yourself and a belief in your training. Interval training on the track can be an important confidence builder.

Interval training is also completely customizable. By juggling Gerschler's five variables, all sorts of training possibilities present themselves. It is an excellent way of adapting the body to stress, since you push, back off, push some more, back off. It also permits you to train at race pace, and it is an excellent way to learn that pace.

After my introduction to interval training in Germany, I experimented a lot with different patterns. My most frequent workouts were 400s (jogging 400s between) or 200s (jogging 200s between). They could be done very neatly on a 400-meter track outdoors or a 200-meter track indoors. (Of course, back then the tracks and repetitions were measured in yards—thus 440 or 220 yards.) Sometimes, I used long repetitions and short intervals, such as 1000s with 200s between, or miles with a quarter-mile jog (or 2-minute walk) between. The latter workout I sometimes did with Tom O'Hara, who set a world record for the mile indoors and ran the 1500 for the United States in the 1964 Tokyo Olympics. It was a workout that O'Hara often did on his easy days, otherwise I never would have been able to stay close to him.

TOO MUCH OF A GOOD THING

At one point, I experimented with megadoses, where I ran 70 × 300 with a 100 jog or 50 × 400 with 30 seconds between. But I found that sometimes the achievement in the workout outweighed achievements in competition.

Eventually, I realized that runners who do too much interval training suffer injuries, possibly from constant stopping and starting and the stress of going around tight turns on a track. Mental fatigue often was as much a problem as physical fatigue. This was during a period when I, and most other distance runners, did *all* our training on a track. The person who did most to influence us was Mihaly Igloi, the Hungarian coach who defected after the 1956 Melbourne Olympics and guided the careers of a group of top Americans, including Jim Beatty, Jim Grelle, and Bob Schul. (Beatty and Grelle were among the top milers in the world in the early 1960s; Schul won the 5000 at the 1964 Toyko Olympics.)

Igloi was a gifted, extremely dedicated coach who nevertheless had a reputation (whether deserved or not) for destroying as many runners as he helped with his intensive training methods. Every workout was an interval workout.

Although I had made major improvements by using interval training, I also was prey to overtraining. Today's system of running away from the track—on roads, in the woods—is superior to what I did decades ago in a frantic effort to succeed. This is why I continue to recommend that you train in various locations, not just on the track.

"The first rule of practice when using genuine interval training," says Brian Mitchell in his article in *Athletics Weekly*, "is don't use it too often, and don't think it will produce all the goods."

Over the decades, I have continued to enjoy occasional interval workouts. My rule for intervals became never more than a dozen, because the purpose for doing such workouts is improving speed as much as stamina. A typical interval workout for me became 10 × 400 with a 200-meter recovery jog between each. I finished refreshed, and I saved the heroics for race weekends.

On the other hand, I never again ran quite as fast as I did after training in Germany's *Schwarzwald*.

QUESTIONS AND ANSWERS

At expos and clinics, as well as on online, I often field questions from runners. Here are some frequently asked questions about interval training and their answers.

Q. What distance should I use for my repeats?

A. The longer the repetition, the greater the development of your aerobic system, which is important for endurance. (Remember, interval refers to the rest or pause in the workout.) The shorter the repetition, the greater the development of your anaerobic system, which is important for speed. You need to develop both systems to run fast. Interval training normally encompasses distances from 200 to 800 meters, but the most commonly used distance is 400 meters, because it's convenient—one lap on a track. Start with 400 meters for your repetitions, and vary the distance as you become more comfortable with interval training. One of my favorite workouts used to be 1000 meters, 200 rest, 200 meters, 200 rest, then repeat.

Some runners favor longer repetitions. Exercise physiologist Jack Daniels, PhD, described having members of his cross-country team at the State University of New York at Cortland doing what he called cruise intervals. These were repetitions as long as 2 miles at slightly slower than race pace, with rest intervals of only 30 to 60 seconds.

Q. How long should I walk or jog during the rest interval?

A. Gerschler controlled the length of his intervals by measuring pulse rate. A runner whose pulse reached 170 to 180 (85 to 90 percent of his MHR) during the repeat would run again when it dropped to approximately 130 (65 to 70 percent of his MHR).

Very fit runners can turn around and start the next repeat within 30 seconds of stopping. I watched two-time Olympic gold-medal winner and former world record holder Sebastian Coe do just that in a workout. Coe ran 20 × 200 in 27 to 28 seconds several weeks before winning the 1500 at the 1984 Los Angeles Olympics. But a more frequent pattern is to jog the same distance during the interval as you run during the repeat. For someone running 400-meter reps, this would mean doing 400-meter jogs in between. After you become more comfortable with this form of training, you may want to cut the distance (thus also the time) of your intervals.

Q. How many repetitions should I run?

A. There are various formulas comparing total volume of running to race or training distance. Ecker suggests $1\frac{1}{2}$ to 3 times race distance (which probably makes more sense for middle-distance runners in track than for distance runners whose race distance is 5K or longer).

Exercise physiologist Jack Daniels, PhD, suggests a cap of 8 percent of weekly training mileage: $1\frac{1}{2}$ miles if you run 20 miles a week; 4 miles if you do 50. Both men are correct, and both are incorrect. Don't put too much faith in formulas—so take the one I am about to give you solely as a recommendation.

A good starting point for runners choosing 400 as the distance for their repetitions is 5. If you can't run 5 reps, you're probably training too fast. A good end point is 10 reps. If you can run more than that, you're probably training too slowly.

Runners choosing 200-meter reps will want to do slightly more; runners choosing 800-meter reps will want to do less. But begin cautiously. Dr. Costill warns that too many runners push hard to make themselves tougher, but instead they push themselves too far. "The danger," he says, "is that they begin to develop poor technique."

Q. How fast should I run my repetitions?

A. Race pace is a convenient and safe measuring point in books and articles, because it compensates for the fact that readers vary greatly, both in their ability to race and in their ability to endure hard training. The best judge of training pace is an experienced coach standing beside the track, and even that coach is probably guessing some of the time. So begin at a pace that is comfortably slower than race pace, progressing to that point and somewhat faster. You probably need to go through several periods of progressive interval training before you begin—and notice that I used the word *begin*—to comprehend how true interval training works.

One frequent recommendation is to choose a pace you would use in a race that is one-half the distance of the event you're training for. If, for instance, your goal is a fast 10K, train at a 5K pace; 5K runners train at a 3K pace, and so forth. Scientists claim that training a bit faster than race pace develops the anaerobic system's buffering capacity—that is, its ability to resist stress. Regardless of scientific explanations, slightly faster than race pace is a good end point for interval training. For those using 400s in their interval training, this would mean running up to 5 seconds per quarter faster than you would in a race.

Q. *What form of rest should I use during the intervals?*

A. There are three types of rest: jogging, walking, or total rest. Actually, there probably is a fourth type: walking and jogging. I once told one of the high school runners I helped coach that he had the fastest move of anyone I had seen from the finish line to a seat in the bleachers beside the track: one and a half strides. He was the Michael Jordan of interval resters. Absolute rest doesn't make sense for interval training. You recover too completely, which defeats the purpose of trying to maintain your pulse rate at a continuously high rate (70 to 90 percent of your MHR) during the workout.

Walking is an effective means of rest for those beginning to use this method of training, although some highly trained runners use very short walks between very intense runs. I sometimes would walk 100, jog 200, and walk 100 while between repetitions. A group of adult runners I trained with at The Bolles School in Jacksonville, Florida, followed this formula, but the most popular (and effective) form of interval rest is jogging the full lap.

Regardless of which kind of rest you choose, be consistent throughout the workout. Don't begin by jogging at a fast pace between repetitions and finish by having to walk. If that happens, you're jogging too fast or running too many repetitions at too fast a pace.

Learn to concentrate in practice, and you can carry that concentration into races.

Q. What can I expect from interval training?

A. In an article in *Runner's World* magazine, Ohio State University's David R. Lamb, PhD, suggested that the biggest benefit was improved running economy. "If you want to improve your economy at your race pace," Dr. Lamb wrote, "you must (train) at or near that pace." Practically every coach agrees with Dr. Lamb.

Interval training also can improve your speed, your endurance, and your pace judgment. But an important, though often overlooked, benefit from interval training is that it improves your ability to concentrate. It is very difficult to run consistent times on a track while allowing your mind to drift (as often happens during long runs). But with intervals you learn to focus your attention on the task at hand. This improved concentration will help with everything you do as a runner.

When I would begin running interval sessions in the spring, I frequently found my mind drifting on the backstretch during 400s, as though on a long run. And usually, I failed to run fast times. As the training period progresses, I discovered I could concentrate for longer periods of time, until finally, I could remain focused for the full lap. And my times would improve, both on the track and in races. I sometimes wonder how much of that improvement was the result of better conditioning and how much was simply from improved concentration. Learn to concentrate in practice, and you can carry that concentration into races.

Q. How much interval training should I do?

A. Dr. Daniels permits his runners to do no more than one interval session a week. Once a week seems to be a good rule. Those of us from previous generations who did interval training more frequently found it difficult to maintain such an intense level of training without injury or overtraining. Believe me: I made a lot of training errors that, when corrected, allowed me to write this book. Today, there are too many other interesting and effective training methods available to distance runners, so why train only one way?

Q. Is there a best time of year, time of week, and time of day for interval training?

A. Yes. More specific answers depend on your goals and level of ability and conditioning. Interval training works very well when you are getting ready to peak for competition, so if you're seeking fast summer times, early spring is a good time to begin. Weather, of course, may dictate when you can interval train. So will availability of training facilities. If you run long (or race on the weekend), you may want to plan your interval session as far from that effort as possible, thus midweek. Interval training also requires at least a 15- to 20-minute warmup (plus a cooldown at the end of the session) and often takes more total time than a distance run. Regarding time of day, do whatever works best for you and fits your life schedule.

Q. Where should I do interval training?

A. The best venue for interval training is the track. Tracks that are 400 meters around are convenient because they usually are marked in 100-, 200-, and 300-meter segments that make it easier to systemize your training. Tracks also offer a form of ambience, since going to the track— driving there, warming up, changing your shoes—signals to your body, "Okay, today's the day we run fast!" Also, training partners often are more easily available at the track. And coaches. But once you learn the basics of interval training and discover how to measure your level of effort by time, pulse, heartrate, or even by your perceived exertion, you can do interval training any place: roads, woods, wherever. At some point, such training blends into fartlek (which I'll cover in Chapter 15), but don't worry about that yet.

Q. How can I guard against overtraining and injuries?

A. Coach Dellinger states that you should be able to run the last repetition at the same pace as the first—or faster. "If it's a real struggle," he warns, "you should start your next workout at a slower pace, or increase the recovery." Dellinger also suggests that runners use training flats, not track spikes, even for running on a track. (The one exception to this would be on a rainy day, when a wet track might be slippery.) There is no foolproof way to avoid overtraining or injury, but if you approach your interval training with the idea that it should be a challenging workout—but not a punishing one—you will find this form of training both more enjoyable and successful.

I also felt that one danger in interval training is the constant stop-and-start. You run a quarter at a fast pace, then slow to jog. At the end of your interval jog, you start to run fast again, and if you are numbers-oriented, maybe you start too fast to shave a few tenths off your time. If you slide gently from one phase to the other, I suspect you can diminish your injury risks. Please be aware that I have no scientific research to prove this theory.

Finally, although interval training is a very precise and scientific means of improving your running ability, don't become bogged down with numbers. "Vary the program," advises Dellinger. "Do different sets of intervals, different distances, and experiment with recovery times." Great advice from a great coach. Although all the experts agree that interval training is one of the most effective types of training devised, it is not the only type, or necessarily the best for you. Use it judiciously if you want to become a fast runner.

CHAPTER FOURTEEN

THE 10K
Training plans for a key racing distance

On an October day, I received a text message from my granddaughter, Holly Higdon, a senior at Saint Mary's College in Notre Dame, Indiana. "Hello," Holly began. "I was thinking about training for a half marathon that takes place next March. I plan to run with two of my friends, who never have run before. Since I haven't run much lately, I thought it might be a good idea to start from the beginning. Should we use one of your novice training programs?"

Oh my goodness: What a delicious message to receive. What grandparent could resist a request—particularly a text message request—from a grandchild asking for advice? In several back-and-forth messages, I elicited from Holly the fact that her chosen race was the Holy Half, an aptly named race organized by students at the University of Notre Dame. The event attracts both students and nonstudents, limited to 1,500 participants on a first-come basis. Holly and her friends had approximately 5 months to prepare. Good for you, Holly, I thought. With that much preparation time, success was almost certainly guaranteed for you and your friends.

I determined that they should start with a short-distance program, which would last about 8 weeks, before plunging into one of my standard 12-week half marathon programs. And what better short-distance program than one for a 10K, which in case you failed to notice is the subject of this very chapter? For Holly and her friends, the 10K could serve as an interim goal en route to her final goal, the Holy Half. (I wondered if I could get the students at Notre Dame to change the name of their race to the Holly Half.)

Holly was far from being a rookie runner. She had run cross-country and track at Michigan City High School. She continued as a cross-country runner her first two years at Saint Mary's. Then, life interfered: Too many conflicts between her music major and afternoon workouts with the team forced her to drop varsity competition. Holly continued to run for pleasure, although her semester abroad in Ireland made it difficult for her to follow a precise schedule. It was now on my shoulders, as grandfather, to reintroduce her to the family sport. I asked her to give me time to think through the particulars of their specific training program, and we agreed to FaceTime later that evening.

After FaceTiming and several more days of planning on my part, I contacted Holly with my plan. I pointed her toward my 10K Novice plan, its main focus getting her back in shape so she could begin half marathon training with a sound base. As for her two friends, not having run before, could they handle a program that has a 3-miler in the first week? Perhaps they could. Perhaps they couldn't. Would they be better backing down to the 5K Novice plan? That would eliminate the advantage of having the three of them—friends, classmates—following the same program. I decided that I would let Holly and her two friends decide which plan to follow. After 8 weeks, Holly and her friends made a smooth transition from the 10K program to the half marathon program.

Other runners might take a different tack when it comes to improving their fitness, improving their speed, and improving their ability to run fast at a multitude of distances. My 10K Intermediate program features 1 day of speedwork. My 10K Advanced program offers 2 speedwork days. Both programs offer more mileage, though the advanced program actually peaks with a 10-mile run in Week 7 before the 10K race in Week 8.

All of my training programs in this book feature a logical progression from a little bit of running to a lot more running, and then often to faster running. In many respects, my 10K programs operate in an important middle ground. If you are a runner whose specialty is endurance, your favorite races being half and full marathon distances, you can drop down to 10K and work on your speed by doing interval training on the track, or tempo runs on the road or in the woods. If your specialty is speed, your favorite races being the 5K, or even shorter distances on the track, you can accept the longer long runs that appear in the 10K training programs to build your endurance.

TRAINING FOR THE 10K

The 10K Novice program differs only slightly from the 8K Novice program presented in Chapter 10. The 10K plan calls for a few extra miles for one of the midweek runs and a few extra miles for the long runs on Sunday, climaxing in Week 7 with 5.5 miles, just short of the 6.2 miles run in the goal 10K. It also offers a few more minutes of cross training on Saturday, but only a few. Rest on Mondays and Fridays. The Wednesday and Thursday workouts for 10K are identical to the Wednesday and Thursday workouts for 8K, but keep in mind you're only adding an extra mile to your race distance. The training should not be that different—or that much more difficult. When I say "run," I mean for you to run at any pace that feels comfortable. If personal plans force you to juggle workouts from one day to another, do so without worry. Here is my 10K training plan for novice runners.

The 10K Novice

WEEK	MON	TUE	WED	THU	FRI	SAT	SUN
1	Rest	2.5 mile run	30 min cross	2 mile run	Rest	40 min cross	3 mile run
2	Rest	2.5 mile run	30 min cross	2 mile run	Rest	40 min cross	3.5 mile run
3	Rest	2.5 mile run	35 min cross	2 mile run	Rest	50 min cross	4 mile run
4	Rest	3 mile run	35 min cross	2 mile run	Rest	50 min cross	4 mile run
5	Rest	3 mile run	40 min cross	2 mile run	Rest	60 min cross	4.5 mile run
6	Rest	3 mile run	40 min cross	2 mile run	Rest	60 min cross	5 mile run
7	Rest	3 mile run	45 min cross	2 mile run	Rest	60 min cross	5.5 mile run
8	Rest	3 mile run	30 min cross	2 mile run	Rest	Rest	10K race

Similarly, the 10K Intermediate schedule differs little from the 8K Intermediate. The main difference between the 10K Intermediate and the 10K Novice is speedwork on Wednesdays: tempo runs on the odd weeks, interval training on the even weeks. Add to that a test 5K race at the end of Week 4. If your local racing schedule fails to provide such a race, moving the practice race to the week before or the week after is an option. Another option would be to run a race at a (slightly) different distance, although I'm not sure picking a race longer than 10K is too great an idea. A third option would be to do a time trial: a one-man or one-woman 5K, just you and your stopwatch over a course that hopefully is somewhat accurate. In a time trial I always find it difficult to match the faster times I find myself capable of running in an actual road race with a medal on the line, but from a training perspective, it probably makes little difference. Going out and blasting a fast workout carries its own rewards.

Please note in the following training plan that in the long runs scheduled for Sundays, in Weeks 6 and 7, you are running farther than you will in your goal 10K race. But as an intermediate runner, there should be no doubt in your mind as to whether you can finish the distance.

The 10K Intermediate

WEEK	MON	TUE	WED	THU	FRI	SAT	SUN
1	3 mile run	3 mile run	35 min tempo run	3 mile run	Rest	60 min cross	4 mile run
2	3 mile run	3.5 mile run	8 × 400 5K pace	4 mile run	Rest	60 min cross	5 mile run
3	3 mile run	4 mile run	40 min tempo run	3 mile run	Rest	60 min cross	6 mile run
4	3 mile run	4.5 mile run	9 × 400 5K pace	4 mile run	Rest	Rest	5K test
5	3 mile run	5.0 mile run	45 min tempo run	3 mile run	Rest	60 min cross	6 mile run
6	3 mile run	5.5 mile run	10 × 400 5K pace	4 mile run	Rest	60 min cross	7 mile run
7	3 mile run	6 mile run	50 min tempo run	4 mile run	Rest	60 min cross	8 mile run
8	3 mile run	3 mile run	5 × 400 5K pace	1-3 mile run	Rest	Rest	8K race

My most difficult program at this distance is the 10K Advanced. Two days of speedwork in the middle of the week, instead of only one. Two test races: a 5K in Week 4 and an 8K in Week 6, if you can find races at those distances on the proper race dates. More mileage, particularly in the weekend long runs, which begin at 6 miles in Week 1 and peak at 10 miles in Week 7, the week before you start tapering for your goal 10K.

The weekend workouts for the advanced program also offer a couple of switches that are designed to make you a faster runner. On the Saturday workout in Week 1, I prescribe a run of 5 miles. But note that two of those miles are to be done at race pace, the pace you hope to achieve in your 10K race. This pattern has the double advantage of raising the degree of difficulty, getting you more out of breath, and teaching you how to pace yourself properly. A too-slow or, even worse, too-fast first mile can waste 8 weeks of hard training. In other words, learning your race pace becomes an important priority.

The 10K Advanced

WEEK	MON	TUE	WED	THU	FRI	SAT	SUN
1	3 mile run	30 min tempo run	6 × 400 mile pace	3 mile run	Rest or 3 mile run	5 mile total 2 mile pace	6 mile run
2	3 mile run	40 min tempo run	7 × 400 mile pace	4 mile run	Rest or 3 mile run	5 mile total 2 mile pace	7 mile run
3	3 mile run	50 min tempo run	8 × 400 mile pace	5 mile run	Rest or 3 mile run	5 mile total 3 mile pace	8 mile run (3/1)
4	3 mile run	30 min tempo run	9 × 400 mile pace	3 mile run	Rest or 3 mile run	Rest	5K test
5	3 mile run	50 min tempo run	10 × 400 mile pace	6 mile run	Rest or 3 mile run	6 mile total 2 mile pace	8 mile run (3/1)
6	3 mile run	30 min tempo run	11 × 400 mile pace	3 mile run	Rest or 3 mile run	Rest	8K test
7	3 mile run	60 min tempo run	12 × 400 mile pace	6 mile run	Rest or 3 mile run	6 mile total 2 mile pace	10 mile run (3/1)
8	3 mile run	30 min tempo run	6 × 400 mile pace	1-3 mile run	Rest or 1-3 mile run	Rest	10K race

Take note 3/1 runs are scheduled for Sunday in Weeks 3, 5, and 7. In an 8-mile run, this would mean running the first three-quarters of the distance (6 miles) at a comfortable pace, then running the final one-quarter of the distance (2 miles) at a faster pace, although not necessarily race pace. Finishing fast in these workouts helps implant in your mind that you can finish fast in the race itself. It's always fun to pass people when in sight of the finish-line clock than it is to be passed because you failed to pace yourself properly.

In terms of running fast and improving your speed, the 10K Advanced program can prove particularly useful. It is short, only 8 weeks long. April and May are great months for running, whether you live in the Sunny South or the Frozen North. The same can be said for September and October. Throw a couple of months of 10K Advanced work into your year's worth of training before starting a longer program in preparation for a fall or a spring marathon. With fewer miles than you would run while training for a marathon, you can focus your attention on speedwork so that you can become a faster runner.

CHAPTER FIFTEEN

SPEED PLAY
Fartlek and tempo training

A woman once passed me toward the end of a 5K race wearing a T-shirt that had on its front, "Fartlek." And on the back, "It's a runner's thing."

Indeed it is, and assuming the woman used that method of training, maybe that's why she sped by me in the closing minutes of the 5K.

Fartlek not only is a runner's thing, it also is a Swedish thing. Fartlek is a Swedish term that roughly translates into "speed play." It was devised roughly 75 years ago by the Swedish Olympic coach Gosta Holmer. If you took repeats, repetitions, intervals, strides, and sprints and dumped them in a bowl and mixed them all together, you would have fartlek. It is a very effective and satisfying form of training when done properly. It's also fun. And although novice runners might be intimidated by a form of training used by Olympic athletes, fartlek actually is quite easy to master. It's user-friendly.

Or so says Lisa Davies, 43, a teaching assistant from Caerphilly, Wales, United Kingdom. Davies loves using fartlek in her training. "I am about as far from being an elite athlete as possible," claims Davies, "yet I find fartlek an easy way to add speed training. Trying to keep track of reps run on a track is a nightmare. I find fartlek much easier to do, using landmarks as my guide: Hard to the next lamppost, then five lampposts, easy."

Along with his training partners, Jason Weller, 43, a manager from Haarlem, the Netherlands, uses fartlek when prepping for a race. "It is way more fun than standard intervals," says Weller.

Cheryl Parrott, 43, a nurse from Kokomo, Indiana, considers fartlek fun. "The irregular pattern is less demanding than scheduled, regimented speed workouts," she claims.

What is fartlek? Why is it better (or more enjoyable) than other forms of speed training? How can you, the runner, incorporate it into your regular training routine?

In an article in *Athletics Journal,* Paul A. Smith described fartlek as "a continuous overdistance run with numerous faster paced interval runs interspersed, until the runner feels tired but not exhausted." Smith claimed that, because fartlek existed in the mind of the runner as a form of play, it deemphasized the feeling or perception of fatigue.

"Fartlek. It's a runner's thing."

Fartlek was first used successfully by the two great Swedish milers of the 1940s, Gundar Hägg and Arne Andersson. It consists of fast, medium, and slow running over a variety of distances, depending on the terrain.

In a typical fartlek workout, you pick some landmark such as a tree or a lampost and sprint to it, then jog until you've recovered. Select another landmark a shorter—or longer—distance away, and run to it at a faster—or slower—pace. The distance and pace are up to you. The most important skill for this drill is listening to your body. Sometimes you may want to jog more. Add some sprints or strides, and maybe even walk, as your mood develops. "An athlete runs as he feels," says coach Bill Dellinger. "A fartlek training session can be the hardest workout a runner does all week, or it can be the easiest." It depends on how you structure the workout and how long you stay out. Dellinger calls fartlek instinctive.

Pam Triest-Hallahan, 55, a teacher from Nashua, New Hampshire, has run fartlek since high school: "I never enjoyed track workouts and find fartlek better since I can do them on trails or on the roads. They are good for learning to focus for a stretch of running which is so important for distance runners."

"In order to be a good distance runner," adds Dellinger, "you have to build strength and endurance, learn race pace, and practice race tactics. Fartlek training can incorporate all of these essential elements into a single workout."

FAST RESULTS, FEW INJURIES

In a *Runner's World* magazine article, Dellinger described a study on the benefits of fartlek versus the benefits of interval training. It included 30 distance runners and was conducted by a graduate student at the University of Oregon. One group ran fartlek, a second group did interval training, and a third group did a combination of both workouts. After a year of training, during which time the runners were tested every 2 weeks, the fartlek group got into shape the slowest and had the poorest early results. But the runners benefited from fewer injuries. The interval group, on the other hand, had the best early marks but also suffered the most injuries. Perhaps because

CHANGING TEMPOS

Fartlek is a form of speed training where you alternate fast and slow running at a variety of distances, almost by instinct. Olympian Bob Kennedy recalls fartlek workouts at Indiana University where four or five runners would run together. Over a distance of 5 miles, each would take a turn dictating pace so the others never knew when to expect what came next. "The pace shifts made you really focus," recalls Kennedy. "The workout simulated what happens in a tough race."

After he graduated, Kennedy had less opportunity to train in a group, but he continued to use fartlek in his training. He suggests that the key to fartlek for individual runners is to have a plan, whether you're running short or long repeats, sprints or tempo. "Know what you're doing," says Kennedy. "If you make your workout up while you're running, it's too easy to sell yourself short." Kennedy believes that the change in tempo is what makes fartlek a valuable workout for building both endurance and speed.

they suffered fewer injuries—and therefore trained more consistently—the fartlek runners began to outperform the interval group toward the end of the study.

But the lesson to be learned came from the third group. This group's performance shone because the runners combined interval training with fartlek. They had better results and fewer injuries. How often in this book so far have I told you that if you want good results (everybody in chorus now), "Do something different!"

Clearly, fartlek can play an effective role in almost any runner's training, particularly in the area of speedwork, if it's combined with other methods.

FARTLEK FOR EVERYONE

Holmer felt that fartlek, done correctly, could be practiced three to five times a week. That's more frequent speedwork than most of us can handle, but let's consider the theories of a respected coach who in his era trained some of the world's most successful middle-distance runners, namely Hägg and Andersson. Their coach recommended running uphill no more than twice a week, preferably on Mondays and Thursdays. "Fartlek brings us back to the games of our childhood," said Holmer. "The runner is forced to explore."

One such explorer is Ellen Boettrich, 65, a retired health specialist from Hilton, New York. In warm weather, Boettrich does what she calls "shade fartlek," running faster in the shade of the trees, then easier in the hot sun.

Holmer operated in an era when competitive runners were only young and highly skilled athletes. (The 5K as a sport-for-all phenomenon hadn't happened yet.) Times have changed, but runners of varied abilities can benefit by including occasional fartlek workouts in their training programs. Please note my use of the word "occasional."

Beginners. Can today's runners of average ability benefit from Holmer's fartlek training? The answer is yes. The Atlanta Track Club, with 100 volunteer coaches (known as Run Leads), offers a series of four In-Training programs that prepare participants for a variety of distances including the 5K, 10K, half marathon, and full marathon. Amy and Andrew Begley became the first full-time coaches for Atlanta Track Club in 2015.

The In-Training participants train on the Piedmont Park Active Oval for many of their workouts. It is an 865 meter crushed gravel loop. "The soft surface is a great place for beginner runners to start to incorporate speed work," says Amy Begley. The participants can do measured distances, or they can use time or partial laps for fartlek training.

Many of the participants are walkers or those who are doing a run/walk program to build up to running. "The biggest lesson the walkers learn in the program," Amy Begley explains, "is that they can do speed work by doing fartlek training of easy-paced walking and speed walking." The Begleys vary the time or distances of the fartlek intervals to work on different paces of walking. "Fartlek training is a great way to get them out of the rut of going the same pace for every workout," says Amy Begley.

Those doing the run/walk program use the fartlek intervals to build up the distance they can run and the speed of their running. Once they are confident in their strength, the participants move to standard distances of intervals. The participants learn pace and get out of their comfort zone by running intervals and staying consistent.

Can new runners who might not have the supervision of a coach benefit from such training? The answer again is yes!

Team members. Different coaches, of course, interpret fartlek in different ways. At the College of the Holy Cross in Worcester, Massachusetts, W. H. "Skip" O'Connor designed a program based on time rather than miles. He also included other elements, which he describes with terms such as bursts, lifts, steady strides, specific hill attacks, fast openers, fast closers, passing pickups, and bolts. Bursts, for example, are 50-yard sprints on a flat area, a half-dozen or so within a 6-minute time span. These are prearranged sprints performed by his entire team at a signal from the leader. Bolts, however, are sudden and unexpected sprints by various individuals, who have been instructed by O'Connor to uncork them several times during the workout.

The self-coached. Russian coach A. Yakimov, writing in *Track Technique,* said he felt that the length of the fast runs, along with the length

It is the intentional variety of fartlek that makes it less stressful.

and form of rest, should be determined according to how the athlete feels physically. The most important ingredient in a successful fartlek workout is constant change of pace. Here is Yakimov's formula:

1. Light running for 6 to 10 minutes as a warmup (A fast, even run for 1000 to 2000 meters)

2. A brisk walk for 5 minutes

3. Light, even running with short accelerations (50 to 60 meters) until you sense some fatigue

4. Light running with the occasional inclusion of four or five fast strides (these are like sudden surges in a race)

5. Fast uphill running for 1 minute

Yakimov stressed that at the end of the workout, you should not feel fatigued, but rather enthused. "Fartlek is not a 'carefree' system as is sometimes thought. It is not to be used only as a rest from hard workouts. It demands no less of physical and psychological strength than any other method."

RUNNING FREE

To simply copy the formulas of Holmer, O'Connor, or Yakimov (or any other coach) would rob fartlek of its greatest advantage—its spirit of free play. Coach Dellinger believes that it is the intentional variety of fartlek that makes it less stressful than other forms of hard running.

The midweek running group led by Angelia Freeman, a program marketing manager from Roseburg, Oregon, alternates between fartlek and sprints. "The ladies learn to feel the difference between giving a burst of speed followed by full recovery. It helps them to realize what it feels like to run on tired legs."

In an article titled "Playing on the Run" in *The Runner* magazine, Merrill Noden described fartlek. "In any interval session—on or off the track—you are measuring two variables: the distance you run and the time it takes," he wrote. "Real fartlek always leaves one or both of these variables unmeasured." As a result, said Noden, it is impossible to pass precise judgment on your effort.

As such, fartlek lends itself as an extremely useful training tool in a cross-country setting, because training venues away from the track are almost always unmarked and undefined. Yes, courses on which runners race frequently come accompanied by mileposts that cannot be totally ignored; but typically, when runners run off-road, whether through the woods or over a golf course, they run free. It becomes easier, then, for terrain to dictate training. A hill encountered becomes an excuse for a short sprint. A smooth straightaway offers an opportunity for a controlled fast run. A patch of soft ground or a stretch of rocky terrain makes it necessary to slow down.

The principles of fartlek do not need to be reserved for special days. You can work fartlek into almost any workout. On your distance days, you can throw in surges or sprints when the spirit moves you.

One winter's day, for example, I was running with Liz Galaviz, the top runner on my cross-country team. It was between seasons. Snow was on the ground, so we ran a 5-mile course through city streets at an undefined pace.

Galaviz was feeling strong, so midway through the run, I found myself hanging on to her fast pace. At an intersection where we normally would have turned right, I pointed her straight up a hill that was 100 to 150 meters in length. We ran the hill side-by-side, and I could hear her breathing become labored. When the hill leveled off and started down, we eased the pace to recover.

"I just did that to be mean," I said.

Galaviz smiled, "I know."

But I did that, as she realized, to toughen her for running short track races later that spring. It was a classic fartlek move, but one that had been inserted within the framework of what had started out as a relatively easy distance run. It was the perfect "speed play."

TEMPO TRAINING

Another form of speed play that began to gain increased acceptance in the early 1990s has various titles, the most popular being tempo training, or the utilization of tempo runs. Unlike fartlek, a tempo run usually consists of a single, continuous surge in the midst of a medium-distance run.

Tempo runs are associated with no specific coach, although the one who probably did the most to publicize this form of training is exercise physiologist Jack Daniels, PhD, who coached the track and cross-country teams at the State University of New York in Cortland. Dr. Daniels wrote an article titled "Cruise Control" in *Runner's World* magazine on what he called tempo running and cruise intervals. The magazine promoted his article on the cover as "The Biggest Training Discovery in 50 Years." Given the popularity of the magazine, you could not have a discussion with a serious runner in the several months after the article appeared without that topic entering the conversation.

TEMPO TIPS

Here are some tips for boosting your anaerobic power with tempo runs.

Hang loose. Structure your tempo runs according to experience, not formulas. Formulas can offer only broad guidelines. Begin by taking a period of time for warm up, and at the end of your workout take a near equal period of time to cool down. In between is the heart of your workout, which should be 20 to 40 minutes.

Run tough. Pick a pace that is comfortably hard. Dr. Daniels and others recommend a pace that is 15 seconds per mile slower than your best 10K pace.

Run solo. You may have trouble finding another runner whose anaerobic threshold matches yours. Even when you can, you should be cautious and run according to your ability. It's too easy to become competitive and push the pace too hard, even in noncompetitive situations.

Forget time. Don't measure your level of intensity by time. It's too easy to fool yourself into thinking you're improving because you did this week's workout faster than last week's. It's too easy to cheat by running the warmup and cooldown sections progressively faster,

Different coaches and exercise physiologists have used different terms to describe this form of training. It has been known as anaerobic threshold training, steady state running, or AT running (I used that latter term most often in the first edition of this book). Peter Snell, PhD, the Olympic champion turned scientist, preferred to call it lactate threshold training. John Babington, coach of three-time world cross-country champion Lynn Jennings, referred to it as up-tempo aerobic running. Ron Gunn, coach at Southwestern Michigan College in Dowagiac, described such workouts as FCRs, for fast continuous runs. In international circles, you may have heard the term Conconis, after Francesco Conconi, PhD, an exercise physiologist from Ferrara, Italy, and adviser for many of country's top distance runners. Today, the term tempo training (and tempo runs) seems to have achieved ascendance.

which defeats the purpose of the workout. The overload principle works with some forms of training, but not here. By jogging easily both at the beginning and at the end of each tempo run, you eliminate any danger of comparing one workout to another.

Run anywhere. The road. The track. The woods. Even on a treadmill in a health club. The important factor is intensity, not how (or where) that intensity is achieved.

Stay smooth. Maintain a steady effort, not a steady speed. If you run out into a headwind, you'll find yourself returning with the wind at your back. Your actual pace should increase, but not your effort. The same is true on hilly courses, where your pulse actually may rise or drop depending on whether you are going uphill or downhill.

Concentrate. You'll find that you are able to run more effectively if you focus on what you are doing. Because of the speed at which you will be moving, tempo runs offer a good opportunity to pay attention to how you can maintain good running form. This body awareness will help you improve your racing later.

Regardless of what you call the workout, it refers to a type of training where you gradually push your pace to a high degree of difficulty and hold it there before relaxing and finally cruising home.

Charting your pace on a graph, you would have a line resembling the classic bell curve that rises, hits a plateau, then declines. The plateau is where the peak training occurs and also where you reach what Dr. Snell identified as your lactate threshold.

Robert Vaughan, PhD, talked about this as the deflection point—the mythical dotted line around 90 percent MHR where your body systems begin to deteriorate. If you run above that dotted line, say at 91 percent, lactic acid begins to accumulate in your muscles and inevitably causes you to crash. But run just below that dotted line, say at 89 percent, and all sorts of marvelous things happen to your level of conditioning.

SECRETS OF THE ANAEROBIC THRESHOLD

Let's refer back to anaerobic threshold as discussed earlier in this book (page 41) and what it means in terms of athletic performance. The term *anaerobic threshold* apparently was coined in 1972 by California physiologist Karl Wasserman, PhD. He measured the blood acidity of individuals undergoing progressively intense exercise and noted that at a certain point, the blood acidity increased suddenly. Dr. Wasserman suggested that this was the anaerobic threshold, the point at which anaerobic metabolism was initiated.

Not all scientists would agree with this assessment today, although in drafting training plans, it becomes convenient to assume that there exists a dotted line above which you do not stay for long if you plan to continue running.

The biochemical mechanisms that produce glycogen, which fuels the muscles, are complex and require various fuel sources. When exercise is moderate, aerobic metabolism predominates. Glycogen is broken down completely. Oxygen combines with freed hydrogen ions to produce water and carbon dioxide, which are easily carried off.

Aerobic is defined as "in the presence of oxygen," meaning that sufficient oxygen is delivered by your cardiovascular system to maintain a steady state of energy production through the breakdown of glycogen. Aerobic activity generally is associated with slow speeds, jogging, or running long distances.

But a new system kicks in after exercise increases in intensity, so the demands for energy exceed the rate at which oxygen can be delivered. Glycogen is broken down anaerobically, but the process is not complete. Lactic acid accumulates, along with free hydrogen ions.

Anaerobic is defined as "without oxygen," meaning that your level of exercise is so intense that your cardiovascular system cannot provide sufficient oxygen for efficient energy production. The waste products cannot be carried away rapidly enough. Consequently, lactic acid accumulates in your muscles and bloodstream and eventually makes it impossible to run farther. Anaerobic activity generally is associated with sprinting or running distances shorter than 1500 meters.

So when does aerobic activity become anaerobic activity? When does a jog become a sprint, at least in perceived effort? Where is the dotted line in running? How can you identify and use this line—or anaerobic threshold—to plan your training runs?

RUN ON THE DOTTED LINE

Presumably, if you were capable of determining your anaerobic threshold, you would have an advantage both in training and in competition. You could train at a pace just below that threshold, permitting you to maximize your effort and energy without suffering from the accumulation of lactic acid.

Could that knowledge also be applied in a race? I'm less convinced of that, since in races between 5K and 10K, well-trained runners eventually must enter the twilight zone above the dotted line to achieve peak performance. If you're doing your job right, you should be near 100 percent of your MHR when you cross the line. An ability to monitor your anaerobic threshold is most useful in practice. But certainly anything that increases body awareness—training or racing—makes you a better runner.

Unfortunately, theory (and what scientists perceive in the laboratory) does not always match reality. In talking about an anaerobic threshold, many runners probably think there is a certain speed (or pace) below which all activity is aerobic and above which all activity is anaerobic. They might visualize 400 meters run in 120 seconds (8-minute pace) as aerobic and in 60 seconds as anaerobic, with the threshold somewhere in between.

This is not true, as David L. Costill, PhD, points out. "In reality, there exists a continuum between aerobic and anaerobic activity. Pure aerobic activity probably does not exist in athletics. It is achieved only at rest or during mild walking. Even in golf, the explosive golf swing is anaerobic."

And even while functioning at a very low energy level—say 50 percent of your MHR—you are exercising both aerobically and anaerobically. You provide oxygen, but not as much as the system demands. As you increase your exercise intensity—going from 60 to 70 to 80 percent or more of your MHR—more of your energy conversion becomes anaerobic. Eventually, you reach that point of muscular breakdown where you can no longer run. Scientists induce this in the laboratory by running a subject on a treadmill, gradually tilting the angle until he no longer can keep pace. For a sprinter struggling down the straightaway in the 400 meters, it certainly seems as though the track is being tilted just before the finish line.

Scientists have studied aerobic energy production since the early 19th century. Since then, aerobic capacity has become relatively easier to measure by standard laboratory techniques and instant digital feedback of analysis like blood and gas exchanges. Although scientists recently have begun to give more attention to anaerobic energy, it is less readily measurable.

One problem with drawing conclusions about the so-called anaerobic threshold from blood and gas measurements is that not all of the action takes place in the blood or immediately affects the oxygen transport systems. The real action occurs in the muscle, and the increase in blood acidity occurs after the fact—how long after, we do not know. It is the acid level in the muscle that affects the muscle's capability to contract—and your ability to run.

The point of this is that the term anaerobic threshold, as it is currently being used by many exercise physiologists and interpreted to the public, is probably a misnomer. To obtain precise measurement, we would need to monitor the acidity within the muscle, no easy task even with the new non-invasive measuring devices available today. Even the smart watch I sometimes wear in training, capable of measuring my pulse and heart rate, allows me to make only an educated guess as to when I am approaching my anaerobic threshold. I assume that dotted line to be at 90 percent of my MHR, 133 out of a max of 150. But my anaerobic threshold could be somewhat higher or somewhat lower, particularly as I age. One factor is my relative fitness level. The anaerobic threshold for an untrained person might be below 50 percent; someone highly trained could redline above 90 percent, although probably not too much beyond.

After a race in Minnesota, I spoke with a runner of average ability from Minneapolis who had visited a fitness center to have his anaerobic threshold tested. Preparing for an important ultramarathon race, he was sparing no expense. The test involved having him pedal on an exercise bicycle while having his air volume and blood lactate monitored. The tester eventually informed the runner that his anaerobic threshold was 130 beats per minute.

That value, 72 percent, seemed rather low for a well-conditioned runner, since he reported his MHR at 180. But the center testers had failed to measure that value; despite the available data, they had merely estimated by using a standard formula. Formulas are fine for predicting average values, but fail to consider specifics unique to an individual athlete. I told the runner that this was a classic case of "garbage in, garbage out." Although the fitness center seemed to be utilizing the latest space-age measuring devices, they lost any chance of a careful measurement of his anaerobic threshold by utilizing a probably flawed estimate of his MHR.

I quizzed the runner further about his training, which he monitored with a smart watch that has a pulse monitor. He and his regular training partner frequently go for 2-hour runs, maintaining a steady pulse rate of 140 to 145, which would mean around 80 percent of maximum. "Then your threshold is probably somewhere around 150," I suggested. I ended by telling the runner he should quit trying to be too scientific and simply train the way he feels.

It's often fun to imbue your training with at least a certain level of pseudoscience.

PULSE TRAINING

Nevertheless, I must confess that it's often fun to imbue your training with at least a certain level of pseudoscience. And measuring your training can provide motivation. At various times, I use a pulse monitor to measure my training, specifically my cardiovascular response to stress.

While I consider pulse monitors to be very useful training tools, most experienced runners probably can tell how well they are running by perceived exertion—by noticing how they feel and by listening to their bodies. Another way to measure effort, of course, is by running over a measured course, but this ignores variables. External factors can render time measurements inaccurate. Hot weather, cold weather, wind, hills, surface conditions—all can make a 1-mile run at an 8-minute pace equal to a much faster effort, even 7:30 or 7:00. One individual coached by Roy Benson had a job with Delta Airlines. She lived in Denver, Colorado, but flew out of Atlanta to Puerto Rico. One day she might be running in dry 40-degree weather at 5,000 feet and the next day running in humid 80-degree weather at sea level. For her, a pulse monitor served very effectively to monitor stress.

You can purchase a pulse monitor or a smart watch capable of tracking your pulse and heart rate at your local running store.

MAXIMUM GAIN

What are the benefits of lactate threshold, or tempo, training? You get maximum gain for minimum damage. According to Dr. Daniels, "Threshold pace training is individualized and adaptable to changes in fitness. It won't cause you to overtrain. It will build your confidence with each workout. And it will produce results, whether you're at the back of the pack, in the middle, or way up front."

How does this training pace compare with race pace? In an article on 10K training in *Running Research News,* Owen Anderson, PhD, an exercise scientist and former columnist for *Runner's World*, identified 5K runners as racing at 95 to 100 percent of MHR, 10K runners at 90 to 92 percent of MHR,

15K and 10-mile runners at 86 percent of MHR, and marathoners at 80 percent of MHR.

Dr. Anderson further suggested that interval training (details of this
intense workout are covered in Chapter 13, starting on page 121) occurs at 90
to 100 percent of MHR. Dr. Anderson concluded that a good pace for anaerobic threshold training might be a pace just a bit slower—about 10 to 15 seconds slower per mile—than 10K pace. Dr. Daniels suggests that in tempo
runs, you should run at the same pace you would run in a race that lasted
approximately an hour. In describing the peak point in tempo runs, I usually
suggest running somewhat slower than your pace in a 10K race. I like to
keep the definition purposely vague, feeling that runners need to learn to
control their own body signals.

Dr. Daniels defines lactate threshold training as a steady, controlled
tempo run that lasts about 20 minutes at threshold pace. He considers a
steady intensity of effort important. "Going too fast is no better than going

20-MINUTE FIX

Twenty minutes is the ideal length of time for the middle
segment—the quality part—of a tempo run, recommends exercise
physiologist Jack Daniels, PhD. Do your normal warmup: 1 to 2
miles jogging, some strides, some stretching. Then, run 20
minutes at a steady pace that Dr. Daniels describes as
"comfortably hard." The pace should raise your pulse to about 90
percent of its maximum, about as hard as you might run in a race
that lasts an hour. Cool down with a 1- to 2-mile jog.

Dr. Daniels says that the workout serves two purposes. "First, it
gives you the feeling of mentally concentrating on an effort for a
prolonged period of time. You learn to endure discomfort. Second,
it benefits you physiologically. Your body becomes better at
clearing lactate. Since you adjust the pace depending on your
ability, the tempo run is adaptable to all runners. "Everybody has
their own threshold pace," says Dr. Daniels. The tempo run can be
done on the track or, preferably, on road or trail courses.

too slow," he says. "A tempo run is hard but controlled. What's important is the intensity, not the time or speed, which can vary depending on the course, the environment, and whether or not the runner is fatigued or well rested."

One important bonus of such running, according to Dr. Daniels, is that it helps improve the runner's ability to concentrate. You don't float along between 80 and 90 percent of your MHR—at least for any appreciable distance—without being focused on what you're doing.

Dr. Daniels suggests a workout structure that involves 20 percent of the total time dedicated to a warmup, 70 percent of the time (20 to 30 minutes) spent as good, hard running, and 10 percent of the total time reserved for a cooldown.

When I include tempo runs in my training schedules for various distances from the 5K to the marathon, both on my Web site and in articles for *Runner's World* magazine, I usually suggest running easily during the first (warmup) phase of the workout, gradually accelerating to near 10K pace—and holding that pace—during the second (threshold) phase, then decelerating back down to easy pace for the third (cooldown) phase. During a typical 45-minute tempo run, the warmup phase might last 10 to 15 minutes, the threshold phase 20 to 25 minutes, and the cooldown phase 5 to 10 minutes. I cite ranges, rather than precise times, for the phases, because tempo runs are best done in the woods or on the roads, where precise distance measurements are not always possible.

One of the appeals of tempo runs is the deliberate vagueness.

Although in a progressive training program I might prescribe tempo runs of 30 to 60 minutes in length from the start to the end of the program, 45 minutes seems about the right length of time for a tempo run, regardless of your relative ability. To do less than 30 minutes doesn't allow sufficient time to squeeze in all the increments. To do more than 60 minutes turns the workout into more of a long-distance run. Forty-five minutes fits well between these two time limits.

One of the appeals of tempo runs is the deliberate vagueness. You don't get too precise with time, length, or pace. In this respect, the tempo run resembles the fartlek workout. Instead, you allow your body to dictate the workout. Admittedly, it does take some experience to read your body signals.

Olympic marathoner Benji Durden uses a different form of this training method while working with runners, both recreational and elite, in Boulder, Colorado. In a very sophisticated 84-week program he designed for my book *How to Train*, Durden prescribed tempo runs that involved both hard and easy runs in the middle of the workout. In one workout that he described as "18 wup/cdn, 2 (5 crisp/3 easy)," he had his runners warm up with 18 minutes at easy pace, run 5 minutes at a crisp or a harder pace, back off for 3 minutes to an easy pace, then run 5 more minutes at a crisp pace before a final 18-minute cooldown. It sounds complicated, but Durden's runners soon figured out what he was talking about. With blended workouts of this sort, the difference blurs between fartlek and tempo training, but what counts is to simply do whatever workout works best for you.

Dr. Costill notes that neither form of workout serves as the be-all and end-all of training for all runners. "All they are," he says, "is a semiquantitative way to have somebody run at a point where they are at a high level of aerobic training."

Regardless of what you call it, I find tempo running, along with fartlek, an enjoyable and effective way to do speedwork.

CHAPTER SIXTEEN

PURE SPEED

Improve your kick

Does a competitor in 5K and 10K events need to worry about pure speed, flat-out speed, absolute speed—or whatever you want to call sprinting as hard as you can? Forget victory at all costs; what about someone whose goals are more modest? If you're only interested in shaving a few minutes off your times for races at different distances, and don't worry about winning races, should you really care how fast you can sprint? Maybe you should; maybe you shouldn't. In all honesty, most midpack runners in road races compete against only their own previous personal achievements.

After all, in races 5K and beyond, victory often goes to the runner capable of controlling and maintaining his speed over the full distance. Milers may rely on their kicks to snatch victory in the last few meters, but 5K runners, such as World and Olympic 5000 meter champion Mo Farah, more often achieve victory by pushing hard in the middle of the race, working at maximum effort, destroying the will of their opponents, and sustaining that tough pace to the end. Or they sit off the backs of the pace leaders, then kick in the final lap.

Regardless of position in the pack, almost any runner who has entered the last stretch and glanced above the finish line to see the digital clock relentlessly ticking away—55 . . . 56 . . . 57 . . . 58 . . . 59—certainly hopes at that moment to have a reasonably good kick.

At the Berlin Marathon one year, I saw exactly that sort of countdown as I neared the finish line. A quick spurt brought me across in a precise 3:09:59. That's far below my PR. Here's some other not-that-impressive numbers. I finished 3,711th overall, 49th in my age group. Big deal, you say. Okay, but when the results booklet eventually arrived by mail, I took pride in the fact that I was the last runner listed among the block of runners finishing between 3:00:00 and 3:10:00. This also allowed me, when asked about my time at Berlin, to say: "Oh, just over 3 hours." I, like most runners, will take my victories where I can get them, thank you.

If working a little harder—or at least fine-tuning your training—might make the difference between clocking 30:00 and 29:59 in your next 10K, would you do it? Sure you would.

Let's face facts: We'd all like a better kick. Regardless of race position, we'd like the ability to take it out of cruise control, when we enter what might be called the kicking zone, those final 100 meters, allowing us to put the pedal to the metal, and raise a cheer from the crowd as we steam past some guy we've been trailing for the last 10 minutes.

Of course, grumblers will say that if you had properly paced yourself during the full length of the race, you would have been able to fully utilize your energy, and not have had anything left for a kick. The goal, it seems, is to finish each race totally spent, knowing that you could not possibly have obtained one more stride from your depleted muscles.

That may be a noteworthy goal for those seeking Olympic medals, but most of us finish races having not quite squeezed the last drop from the lemon. Even the best of us operate somewhere around the 98th or 99th percentile when it comes to extracting energy. During a career that has spanned a half-dozen decades, I figure I've had maybe three or four perfect races— yes, absolutely *perfect*—when I could not possibly have run a tenth of a second faster. Usually, some reserve remains, both psychological and physical.

Let's face facts: We'd all like a better kick.

Most of us can reach down and find an untapped reserve. By driving our arms, by lifting our knees, we can move fast at the finish. In doing so, we are not necessarily utilizing energy or activating muscles that might have better been used earlier. We are actually tapping different energy systems and utilizing different muscles—sprinter's muscles—that otherwise go unused.

REACHING TOP SPEED

Apart from any advantage in having pure speed to utilize in the kicking zone, such speed is important to use throughout the length of your race. If you can teach yourself to be a better sprinter and to be a more efficient and economical runner, you will run faster throughout the entire race, not just at the end.

One way to improve pure speed is to start with the three S's: sprints, strides, and surges. Let me explain these terms.

Sprints. A sprint usually means just that: an all-out sprint for as long as you can hold it, or want to hold it. Sprinters, such as the great Olympic Gold Medalist Usain Bolt from Jamaica, usually reach top speed at about 60 meters into a 100-meter dash, then merely maintain that speed until they hit the finish line. Among 200-meter runners, the winner is not always the fastest, but rather the one who slows the least after reaching top speed. That was Olympic Gold Medalist Carl Lewis's skill. Scientists suggest that 300 meters is about as far as humans can sprint at full speed without beginning to slow down significantly. If you watched Olympic Gold Medalist Michael Johnson set the world record of 43.18 for 400 meters at the 1999 World Track and Field Championships, though, you might question that scientific opinion. Certain truly gifted runners—Bolt, Lewis, Johnson—sometimes seem to attain a level of performance above and beyond normal human ability.

Strides. A stride is somewhat slower than a sprint. Some strides can be very fast, where the runner gradually accelerates and actually reaches top speed during at least a brief portion of the

INTENSITY

Kenneth Sparks, PhD, an exercise physiologist at Cleveland State University, believes that the key to success in any training session is intensity. "The important Swedish research with the Kenyans suggests that's one reason why they run so fast: They train at a higher percentage of their capacity.

"The LSD (long slow distance) movement hurt us. People got the idea that they could go for long, slow runs and benefit. I don't think that's true. I do long runs at a quality pace—or shorten the runs to 9 to 10 miles. It does take more out of you, and you have to be more careful as you get older, so you program in plenty of rest. But keep the quality up."

distance. Other strides can be relatively slow, since you can run no faster than your race pace and still call it a stride. Strides are often used for recovery on easy days. Sprints and strides are variations on the same theme. Different coaches might define them differently, but both are runs of short distances: a straightaway on a track or a short fairway on a golf course (about 100 meters). One is simply slower than the other.

Surges. A surge is a fast burst—a sprint or stride thrown into the middle of a distance workout. Fartlek, described in Chapter 15, consists of a series of surges. Tempo runs, however, would not qualify under this category, because usually they feature only a single (and gradual) acceleration. Top runners often use midrace surges as strategic strikes, launched in an effort to break away from the competition.

Are you confused? That's understandable, because the difference between the three S's is not great. They're all variations on the same speedwork theme. They all are, however, important tools that can be utilized to improve your speed. Let's discuss sprints, strides, and surges at somewhat greater length.

STRESSING THE MUSCLES

There is a subtle difference between sprints and the two forms of speedwork covered in previous chapters: repeats and interval training. When I run repeats, I run nearly flat-out, fully anaerobic, but with maximum rest. In interval training, I usually run under control but with less rest, doing a mixture of anaerobic and aerobic work.

A sprint is running flat-out, but over a shorter distance, so as to stress (and train) the muscles more than the cardiovascular system. Sprints, like repeats, are totally anaerobic, although if enough of them are run with jogging in between, the effect may be similar to that of interval training. At one point in my career, I ran sprint workouts that hit a peak at 50 × 100 meters. Utterly foolish, I realized afterward. I could identify no benefits from that particular workout, so never did it again. The workout defeated the purpose of sprints, which, at least the way I did them later, occupied a middle ground between repeats and intervals.

What's the scientific rationale for going faster in practice than you would in a race? I asked that question to David L. Costill, PhD.

Dr. Costill mentioned technique—the ability to run efficiently at a very fast pace—then added, "I've never been convinced that you develop greater energy production for the anaerobic system by doing anaerobic training. That system can be taught to work quite well when only moderately trained, such as through interval training. The real advantage of running faster is that you get stronger."

Most track athletes run sprints on the track. They sometimes call them straightaways, because a convenient way to do them is to sprint one straightaway, jog easily around the turn, and then sprint the next straightaway. Other runners prefer to walk between sprints. They will walk, stop, turn around, walk, jog, and sprint back in the other direction. Or they walk back to where they started and sprint back in the same direction. When I included sprints in my warmup before a track race or even a road race, I usually stopped and walked back halfway, then jogged to where I planned to start my next sprint. It's a matter of personal preference and convenience as to how and where you run your sprints.

Usually, I prefer running sprints on soft surfaces. If the track surface is hard asphalt, which is what you'll find at most high school tracks, you may be better off running your sprints on the grass inside the track. But test the softness and smoothness of any surface before you run hard on it. Football fields often take a lot of abuse. For sprinters, an uneven surface can be an ankle injury waiting to happen.

More often, I use the fairway of a golf course. I live a half-mile from Long Beach Country Club, a private club that, fortunately, does not have a fence around it. During summer months, I arrive early in the morning before the golfers, sometimes even before sunrise. It's a cool, pleasant part of the day. There are several fairways that I favor for sprints, depending on where the greenkeepers are mowing that morning.

I prefer running sprints on soft surfaces.

I run from tree to tree rather than any specific distance. The actual details are irrelevant. Time doesn't matter. Distance doesn't matter. Regardless of where you run your sprints, on a golf course or at the track, I consider it useless to time yourself for any distance shorter than 200 meters. Time differences in tenths of a second from one sprint to another mean little. If you're timing yourself, you're diverting your concentration by clicking your watch on and off. Focus your attention on running as swiftly and smoothly as you can for as far as you can, and worry about times at some other point in your training.

GETTING SPRINTS AND STRIDES RIGHT

How far should you run your sprints? Distance is not that important, but I recommend confining yourself to approximately 50 to 150 meters—about the length of a track straightaway, or a fraction of a golf fairway. If you run much farther, you're training for something other than pure speed. You begin to train for speed endurance, the ability to maintain speed rather than to increase it. Each form of training has a place in a well-balanced training schedule.

When I was coached by two-time Olympian Fred Wilt, he told me that distance runners should run sprints at least once a week for three reasons.

1. To develop muscular strength

2. To accustom the cardiovascular system to tolerate a much higher level of effort than normally encountered at race pace

3. To develop anaerobic endurance

I still consider Fred's reasoning to be sound. Of the three reasons he suggested, I consider developing strength to be the most important. Dr. Costill agrees. "Strength equals speed," he says.

DOES SPEEDWORK INCREASE INJURY?

At the University of Otago in New Zealand, William G. Hopkins, assisted by David G. Hewson, studied 350 runners (118 female, 232 male) over a period of 2 years. The runners ranged in ability from elite to average.

By means of questionnaires, Hopkins and Hewson looked at four phases of the runners' training: buildup, precompetition, competition, and postcompetitition. They then compared that data with how often the runners lost days to overtraining, injury, or illness.

What caused runners to lose time due to injury? Whether or not they stretched, the training surfaces on which they ran, nor their age, sex, or race history directly affected injuries. Those getting hurt most often were those who did extra strength training during the precompetition phase and those who did long running at a pace slower than race pace during all phases of their training. Those hurt least were those who included fast running during their buildup as well as precompetition phase.

Hopkins deduced that it was unwise to skip speedwork for fear of injury. In fact, he recommended that you keep your training pace race-specific. "The take-home message," says Hopkins, "is to cut back miles, but to retain high-intensity work."

When sprinting, one variation Wilt suggested was to gradually acceler- ate to top speed at around 50 or 60 meters, then to gradually decelerate. You can do this when running either sprints or strides. Try it and see how it feels.

I used strides as therapeutic repair work, sometimes after a long workout or on what I would classify as an easy day. To me, strides were another form of stretching. I also used strides as part of my warmup before racing or before serious speedwork sessions of repeats or interval training. If I'm run- ning eight straightaways as part of a warmup, the first three or four will be strides (gradually increasing in tempo), with one or two full sprints before closing with one or two strides. Yes, I know. You're probably having a hard time keeping sprints and strides straight in your mind. It takes time, but eventually you can develop the speed routine that works best for you.

A DRILL FOR RECOVERY

There are other benefits to this type of training. Many distance runners include long runs as part of their regular training. We're out every weekend running anywhere from 10 to 20 miles. That's what makes us strong, but often, running a long, slow distance leaves your legs stiff and tight. That's one reason why distance runners lose flexibility, an essential component for running fast. As part of my recovery from long distance, I often breezed through a short, second workout later in the day that consisted mainly of strides. Now that I'm older (and perhaps wiser), I'll run a workout of strides later in the week as well.

One of the main reasons I run strides is to undo some of the damage, such as stiffness, that results from my long or hard workouts and to prepare myself for further fast training.

Remember that while sprints build strength and speed, strides serve best for recovery. A session of easy-flowing strides will set you up to run harder, faster workouts in the days or weeks to come. And those designated tough workouts will build strength and speed.

For me, a typical recovery workout featuring strides would be to jog from my home to the golf course, taking a slightly extended route so that I arrive there after covering about 1 mile. I stretch under an evergreen tree beside the first fairway, dangling from a low branch as one of my stretches. Then, I jog over to the 18th fairway, where I stride through eight or more 130-yarders (tree to tree). Following that, I jog home by a slightly longer route. This gives me a workout of maybe 3 miles. It doesn't look overly impressive in my training log, but it's good for my body.

Generally, the first stride is little more than a bowlegged shuffle as I work out the kinks from my previous hard workouts. More often, I walk rather than jog between. By the time I have completed eight strides, I usually am able to run a respectably fast pace, though still not a sprint. I avoid punishing myself and quit while I still feel good. Usually, as I jog back home, I run much more relaxed than I did on the way out. I enjoy the sunrise. I wave at the greenkeepers, who wave back. I finish refreshed. There's nothing scientific about the workout, but it feels good.

A GREAT WARM-UP

Strides also form part of my prerace warm-up, which usually begins with a mile or two of jogging. After some relaxed stretching, I run two to four strides of 75 meters or so at a pace that seems to feel comfortable. After more jogging, I am ready to race. This warmup is a holdover from my track days, and it works for me.

Exercise physiologist Jack Daniels, PhD, is among the respected coaches and experts who recommend strides as an important element of training on so-called easy days. Exercise scientist Owen Anderson, PhD, when discussing Dr. Daniels's training recommendations in his publication *Running Research News,* described a method of doing strides.

Midway through or at the end of your easy run, run for about 100 meters at close to your mile pace. (Don't sprint; try to run comfortably.) Following each stride, jog lightly for 15 to 20 seconds before commencing the next stride. After five strides have been completed, walk around for a couple of minutes until you feel completely rested and recovered, and then do a second set of five strides to finish your striding for the day. The purpose for strides is to reinforce the mechanics of race pace (you get 10 chances to run at race speed) and perk up what might be a boring training day. At first, try doing strides on one or two of your easy training days each week; if all goes well, you can increase the number of days you do strides.

I will also use strides as part of my prerace taper, particularly if the race is a marathon. In designing tapering programs for the marathon, I usually recommend that 2 of the last 3 days involve complete rest with about 2 miles of running on the remaining day of the taper. Because we all are creatures of different habits, I say that I don't care on which days you rest and on which days you run. My preference, however, is to run easily on the day

WHY SHORT SPRINTS?

When you say "speedwork," the very word scares a lot of runners. But this important form of training does not need to be too fast, nor too hard. Particularly for adult runners, coach Roy Benson recommends what he calls "aerobic" intervals.

Benson identifies these as short pickups of no more than 20 seconds that you incorporate into your training program at various times of the year. "If you do only slow distance, particularly during your base training phase," says Benson, "you lose biomechanical efficiency. Short sprints can help you balance strength and flexibility and improve leg coordination."

The effort should be fast but easy. "Think legs, not lungs," Benson advises. "The idea is to use as big a range of motion with as rapid a turnover as possible, but for a short enough distance so that you never huff and puff. If you do pickups longer than 20 seconds, they should be run at no more than 80 percent effort. That is just at the top of your aerobic zone and all the higher you want to go."

before the marathon. In other words, rest Thursday and Friday and run Saturday before a Sunday marathon.

Many runners are surprised when they see my schedules with a 2-mile workout on Saturday. "Won't that tire me out?" they ask. Possibly, but more important, an easy run of about that length will help loosen you up, particularly if you spent the day before cooped up in an airplane or car. And what is at the heart of that recommended 2-mile workout the day before? You guessed it: strides! Before the Boston Marathon, I would usually jog from my hotel near the finish line on Boylston Street to the Charles River (a distance of about a mile), do three or four strides on a grassy area, then jog back. It's what I needed to get race-ready. Many marathoners refer to this as a shakeout run because it helps to get rid of any prerace jitters and anxiety.

Learning to run strides is simple. It took about 15 seconds of instruction for me to teach a new member of my cross-country team how to run strides. Experiment with this form of speed training and see how easy it is.

Research suggests that lactic acid buildup in the muscles is insignificant in the first 20 seconds of fast running, but it almost quadruples between 20 and 30 seconds. That causes eccentric contractions to begin and forces your muscles to extend while still tight. "You tie up, and that's what we try to avoid by stopping short of maximum effort," says Benson. "Aerobic speedwork can be easy if you do it correctly."

A simple and effective way to do this workout is at the track: sprinting the straightaways, jogging the turns. Or do stopwatch fartlek. Run hard (without straining) for 20 seconds on your watch, then jog for the remainder of the minute. In other words, go 20 seconds hard, 40 seconds easy.

Or you can throw speed bursts into the middle of your long runs. About two-thirds of the way through a 6-mile run, start doing pickups. Cover 1 to 1½ miles this way. "But keep the effort easy," warns Benson. "Don't force yourself, or you defeat the purpose."

BREAK AWAY FOR BETTER PERFORMANCE

"Surges" may be the third "S," but they fit uncomfortably beside sprints and strides. Some runners might argue that surges do not qualify as pure speed, and they probably are right—except that while you are surging, you usually are moving at a very fast pace.

What are surges? They are fast sprints thrown into the middle of a long run. Coach Ron Gunn at Southwestern Michigan College in Dowagiac used to refer to surges as break 'em drills, since by surging in the middle of a race, you often can break away from your opponent. He had his runners wait until the final third of a workout before doing surges. "If they do them too early, you'll lose them for the rest of the run," says Gunn.

I often include surges in the middle of a hard, fast run. For example, while doing a fast 6-miler, I might begin at a 9-minute mile pace. But after a few miles of gradual acceleration, I'll reach a steady pace near 8 minutes, holding it for several miles. During the middle of this workout, if I'm feeling strong, I might attempt several surges—I pick up the pace to faster than 7 minutes, hold it for several hundred yards, then ease slightly, only to surge again. Obviously, the pace increment for different runners would vary according to ability. A world-class runner might surge to a near 4-minute-mile pace; most of the rest of us would be surging considerably slower.

On other occasions, I will run long surges, changing pace several times during a run of anywhere up to an hour's duration. One example is when I used to run with my high school cross-country team in the Indiana Dunes State Park over a figure-eight course that included what we called the ridge trail, a wooded bluff high over the beach. We would begin by running about 10 minutes until we reached a point in the woods where we would stop and stretch. Then we headed up onto the ridge. The trail wound back and forth, dipping and diving, forcing runners to make constant surges, a series of sprints or strides thrown into the middle of what is essentially a long run. At the end of the ridge, we would relax, coast, regroup, and let gravity carry us down a sand dune. We would back off the pace for a mile or so before turning onto a trail and boardwalk that crossed a swamp, which coaxed us into a long surge before returning to our starting point.

> *Knowing how and when to surge can offer a tactical edge.*

Wait a minute, you say. Weren't you training speed endurance rather than pure speed? Many forms of speed training overlap. They lead into each other. They complement each other. In actuality, we trained using a blend of repeats and interval training. The easy run between ridge and swamp served as our interval. It's also a form of fartlek. Don't get hung up on terms. Sometimes, you want to go out and try different forms of speedwork just for variety and to feel the wind in your hair without worrying about whether it improves your performance.

For elite athletes, such as Olympic gold medalist Mo Farah or Olympic silver medalist Galen Rupp, who are trying to break their rivals in the middle of a 5000-meter race, knowing how and when to surge can offer a tactical edge. Similarly, a surge can also assist a high school cross-country runner trying to move from 57th to 56th place at the state championships.

So, do surges make sense for adult fitness runners? Granted, if you surge more than once or twice in the middle of a marathon, you may never make it past 20 miles. But surges and the other forms of speedwork described in this chapter make sense for two reasons. One, practicing surges will improve your basic speed, which can translate to improved performance. Two, being able to change pace midrace can help get you out of a rut, or put you back on pace, which can result in a faster time. Don't overlook the benefits of learning how to run fast.

And when you see that digital clock over the finish line relentlessly ticking away—55 . . . 56 . . . 57 . . . 58 . . . 59—you'll be glad you have a kick.

CHAPTER SEVENTEEN

DYNAMIC FLEXIBILITY

Speed in motion

Roy Benson, an Amelia Island, Florida, fitness consultant and former University of Florida track coach, stands before a group of several hundred teenagers jammed into the bleachers of a gymnasium in Asheville, North Carolina. They are high school cross-country runners spending a week at his summer running camp to become better runners. With the week of hard training at Benson's camp, plus the knowledge gained, they hope to return home with skills not possessed by their rivals.

You may wonder what you can learn from a group of high school runners. Plenty. Coach Benson's advice applies to any runner hoping to learn how to run fast.

Today's lesson is dynamic flexibility—although Benson does not call it by that name, nor does he use terms like plyometrics, ballistic stretching, speed drills, or bounding drills. Different coaches favor different terms. Regardless, dynamic flexibility is a form of stretching—a means of getting loose—that involves continuous movement, as opposed to the static nature of regular stretching.

At his camp, Benson offers what he describes as "learn-by-doing drills." He promises the runners, "These drills are going to teach you how to get stronger, how to be more flexible, how to be more coordinated." Soon, he has them out of the bleachers and lined up facing him on the wide side of the gym.

Benson concedes that one way for runners to improve their speed is to increase their running distance. "If you're running 20 miles a week, I'll guarantee that if you can move up to 40, you'll run faster." That is a basic fact proved by not thousands, but millions, of runners at the front of the pack, at the back of the pack, and at every point between.

But one problem as runners increase distance, he continues, is that they often decrease flexibility. "The first thing that happens is that your hamstrings get tight, because you're using this short stride. Your calves get tight, your shins get tight, your quads get tight. You develop inflexibility, resulting in a shorter and shorter range of motion, and pretty soon, you can't run as fast." Benson states that runners must continue to fight this tightening process by using flexibility drills.

Not just static stretching: flexibility drills.

Another factor, Benson explains, is that by not working the muscles used when you run fast, those muscles weaken and compound the problem. Finally, says Benson, runners who run long also run very erect, landing toward the rear of their feet, on their heels. That may be an economical way to run distance, but not to run fast. For speed, runners need to learn to land farther forward on their feet—more midfoot, toward their toes.

Benson asks those at his camp to run in place. Soon the gym thunders with the sound of thumping shoes.

This is the first step in learning flexibility: employing simple movements that will help you loosen up. There are, of course, different approaches. In fact, a generation of runners has been taught that the best way is to stretch in a static position. "Don't bounce!" is a warning offered by almost every stretching expert, including Bob Anderson, author of a bestselling book on that subject.

Anderson writes in the book *Stretching*, "Holding a stretch as far as you can go or bouncing up and down strains the muscles and activates the stretch reflex. These harmful methods cause pain, as well as physical damage due to the microscopic tearing of muscle fibers."

That's great advice, but static stretching is not the only way to loosen up. Fast running is another way. Simply by sprinting out and lengthening your stride (the sprints, strides, and surges discussed in Chapter 16), you stretch your muscles. Of course, you have to be loose to run fast, so it becomes a question of which comes first, the chicken or the egg—the stretch or the stride? The truth is that dynamic flexibility drills do not replace static stretching. Rather, they often work well together.

HIGH KNEES

"Stop!" Benson yells out to his class, and he asks how many were landing on their heels. Nobody raises a hand. Benson nods and explains that it is impossible to run in place landing on your heels.

Benson again asks them to run in place—but to now begin moving forward gradually, across the gym. The campers comply and, in so doing, learn one of the first drills, what in an article I wrote many years ago for *The Runner* magazine I dubbed "high knees." In this drill, runners thrust their knees upward vigorously, counterbalancing with powerful arm pumps. It's more like sprinting in place than running in place.

As the campers move from one side of the gym to the other, Benson instructs, "Stay up on your toes! Get that feel. Feel yourself coming down on your midfoot, the ball of your foot. That's the feeling you want when you run fast."

To emphasize the high-knee aspect of the drill, Benson next has the high schoolers hold their hands out in front of them, just higher than their knees. Jogging back across the floor, they hit their hands with their knees, gradually raising their hands and lifting their knees to waist height.

"One of the side benefits of these drills is to turn you into better athletes," he says. "We want to make you feel more comfortable and coordinated when you sprint." Benson notes that high-knee drills are good for strengthening the hip flexors, which he identifies as the most important running muscles in your body. "The only way you strengthen your hip flexors," he says, "is to run up hills or stadium steps, or do speedwork—or do drills such as this." He advises running drills when you're fresh, not when you're fatigued from a hard workout. That being the case, for those following one of my training programs, dynamic flexibility drills are best done on the easy days, when I suggest going for an easy run of 3 miles or so.

A variation on high knees is a less dynamic drill I call the drum major. I used it with my cross-country teams. Instead of running in place, it's more like walking in place. The motion is the same. Rise up on one toe, thrusting the opposite knee as high up toward your chest as possible, using a vigorous arm pump to achieve this. But you walk, rather than jog or run. You don't leave the ground, so it's a safe drill to do if you're recovering from a minor injury. I also recommend the drum major as a good introductory drill for older runners who have just begun to get acquainted with dynamic flexibility drills in an attempt to improve their running.

"One of the side benefits of these drills is to turn you into better athletes."

Some risk does accompany drills that involve some form of bounding, particularly for those with an insufficient training base or those like me who have passed their 40th birthday. Nevertheless, masters or beginning runners can start with the drum major as a prelude to high knees. But don't abandon it once you've learned the more dynamic drills. It remains a good flexibility drill for all ages and levels.

A complementary static exercise to high knees or the drum major is the knee pull. Stand in place, and with both hands, pull one knee to your chest, stretching your hamstring. Still another stretching variation is to do this while lying on your back. While warming up before a race, I sometimes use all three drills—high knees, drum major, and the knee pull—to loosen my muscles.

I also use the knee pull while soaking in a hot whirlpool. It's one of my favorite stretches, mainly because I constantly must fight the tendency of my hamstrings to tighten during long runs. Most distance runners have tight hamstrings; they come with the territory. It's one reason why we have trouble touching our toes.

HIGH HEELS

High knees is perhaps the easiest flexibility drill to learn and practice, and once his students have a handle on it Benson moves to the next drill, what he calls the fanny-flicker and what I call high heels. Coaches sometimes call it the butt-kicker. I also sometimes refer to it as the glute-kicker, as in gluteus maximus, your butt muscle.

Benson begins by walking his group through the drill on their toes. "As you go farther and farther, lift your heels higher and higher, until you're kicking your fanny." Leaning forward makes the exercise easier to learn, although I recommend an upright posture for more practiced butt-kickers. Once Benson's campers learn the movement in slow motion, he brings them butt-kicking back across the gym. "Nice and slowly," says Benson. "Short steps. The minute you try to go fast, it gets too challenging and you fall apart. Short steps. *Flick! Flick! Flick!*"

Benson nudges me and points toward two girls—sprinters, as it turns out. "Watch their kick," says Benson. "They get perfect full extension across the front of their ankles. Their toes point. The classic back kick. That, to me, is the secret of speed."

Indeed, one way to judge a runner's speed is by watching him or her do these drills. On one of my cross-country teams, two runners clearly drilled better than the others. Had you sent that team across the grass in one of the above drills, you would immediately have noticed Don Pearce and Liz Galaviz. Pearce qualified for the state championships in his junior and senior years by running the 800 meters in 1:57. Galaviz, a talented sophomore, was the best half-miler on the girls' squad; that year, she ran 2:32 to qualify for sectionals.

Ironically, Pearce was perhaps the least flexible runner on the team, so static stretching was very difficult for him. And because he didn't like to be seen doing poorly in any activity, he did his stretching routine very reluctantly. If Pearce had a fault (shared by many runners), it was his tendency to rely on his natural ability. Would he have become an even faster runner had he paid more attention to improving his flexibility? I'm inclined to think so, although scientific research offers no proof.

Coach Benson explains to his class that the high heels drill works well for stretching the hamstrings, but it is particularly effective for stretching the quadriceps. "You have to relax your quads to get that heel up," he instructs.

For older, beginning, or injured runners, walking in place with the high-heel motion works quite nicely. As a complementary static stretch for this drill, try the heel hold. Use one hand to balance yourself on a stationary object and the other to pull one heel up toward your butt. For those of you reading this book who are new to this sport, if you go to almost any road race, you will notice many before the start using high heel stretches to both loosen their muscles and quell their nervousness.

SKIPPING

High knees and high heels are great for beginners because they require relatively little skill or initial flexibility. Benson's next set of drills, which involves skipping, is trickier. He teaches two variations: skipping for height (trying to go as high as you can) and skipping for distance (trying to cover as much ground as possible).

Both varieties are extremely dynamic and involve all of the major muscles used in running fast. Thus, skipping is the heart of dynamic flexibility. It is essential that you become loose enough to do this dynamic exercise, just as you should with static stretching, high knees, and high heels. There is no single stretch that complements skipping, although it might be said that all stretches do just that.

Many runners have difficulty learning skipping drills at first, even though most of us skipped naturally as young children. Perhaps it's just a matter of practicing it again. When my oldest son, Kevin, appeared for cross-country practice at Indiana University, he kept getting his legs crossed when coach Sam Bell taught the team the drill. Kevin eventually went behind the dormitory one Sunday morning and practiced skipping until he learned the rhythm. If you have problems learning to skip again, don't feel embarrassed. With some practice, you can master this skill. Kevin did, and it helped him finish the season as the second-fastest runner on the Hoosier team that won the Big Ten title and placed eighth at the NCAA championships. The only runner faster than him was Olympian Jim Spivey.

> *Many runners have difficulty learning skipping drills at first.*

As Benson sends his campers skipping across the gym, sure enough, one lad keeps getting legs and arms tangled. Arm movements in skipping are like arm movements in running or walking: the left arm comes up as the right knee comes up, and so forth. But this camper keeps getting his left arm and left knee up together, until finally everything falls apart. Benson sends him back and forth across the floor several times, but the camper just can't seem to pick up the right rhythm.

It's not easy. For this reason, Benson instructs his students on the technique of skipping. "To skip, you must be coordinated. You start skipping with high knees, stay relaxed, and slowly bring your arms in like a sprinter. Arms are straight, pointing down the track, not across your body. You want to have straight hands, up about jaw height, so you're pumping your arms, getting up in the air. I want to see you hanging like Michael Jordan! Pump your arms. Elbows go as high as possible in the back. That helps you push harder against the ground with that opposite toe. Then come up in the front with a short punching motion to help you lift in the air. Now let's try it slowly. Everybody together, doing a little skip with your arms up. Get those knees high! Hang up there!"

Admittedly, skipping is not easy to explain—or teach. And it was not easy for me to write the previous paragraphs with any hope that everyone would understand what I just had written. When it comes to skipping, you just do it. If you think too much about what you're doing, it may confuse you more. One way to learn to skip is to make very slow and short movements at first: Skip a few inches forward on one foot, then the other. Hold both hands in front of you for balance. Gradually let your hands counterbalance your foot movements. Then stretch out. Once you learn to skip, you'll be amazed how simple—and fun—the exercise becomes.

As I mentioned earlier, there are two variations on the skipping drill: skipping for height and skipping for distance.

Skipping for height is akin to high knees. You move forward gradually, concentrating on getting high off the ground. Accentuate your knee rise. Counterbalance with your arms. As one knee comes up high, the opposite arm thrusts skyward in a palm-open movement. Don't try to cover too much ground. When my team did skipping for height, I would yell at any of my runners who tried to "win" the drill by moving ahead of the others. Getting up in the air is more important than how fast or how far you go. Indeed, those doing the best job with this exercise are often in the back rather than the front.

Skipping for distance is similar in its movements, only now you try to cover distance horizontally rather than vertically. The knees and arms still come up high, but movement is more forward. I discouraged those who tried to "win" the drill, since moving forward too rapidly makes the skipping too difficult to maintain.

Skipping drills are best conducted on smooth, soft surfaces. Football fields are sometimes too lumpy for safe practice of this or any of the other drills noted in this chapter. The tracks around them often are too hard. Basketball courts are okay, since the wood floor offers some bounce. The perfect surface is the fairway of a golf course—if you can avoid being evicted by the greenkeepers or hit on the head by a nine-iron shot, purposely aimed. I also enjoy throwing a few skips into my warmups before a race, mostly just for the fun of it. It looks so quirky that other runners smile when they see me doing it.

TOE WALK

As his campers skip back and forth across the gym floor, Benson talks to me about speed. "When you go to sprint, you don't care about economy. You don't care how smooth and relaxed you are. You want to be powerful, dynamic. You pump your arms to make your strides go faster. You turn over quicker. That way, you'll really take off."

Benson has one final drill to teach his campers: the toe walk, a less dynamic variation of the drum major, discussed earlier. It's a good exercise for calf muscles—and a simple one. All you need to do is walk forward and accentuate your toe push-off: rolling up and over on the toes of the feet. "Way up on your toes," says Benson. "Don't bounce. Walk. Stay up on your toes. Feel your calves tightening. You're building power, strength, explosion."

Having used nearly an hour to teach four simple drills (high knees, high heels, skipping for height and for distance, and toe walks), Benson releases the group to its next activities. Had he the time or the inclination, Benson could have offered several additional speed drills.

Any time you use different or untrained muscles, you probably will feel sore.

Beginning runners may feel as though they crash-landed at the bottom of the cliff the day after their first dynamic flexibility drills. Any time you use different or untrained muscles, you probably will feel sore for 24 to 72 hours afterward, and it makes little difference how otherwise well-trained you are as a runner. The same would happen if you switched suddenly to cycling or skiing or tennis. For this reason, introduce bounding drills very gradually into your program. Begin with only one or two drills and minimal repetitions. Do them on your easy days. Gradually introduce additional drills and increase the number of repetitions. You will avoid both discomfort and the increased risk of injury that comes as the price for wanting to run fast.

FAST FEET

One additional drill that I used with my teams is fast feet. It's one that I learned from the late University of Oregon coach Bill Bowerman. I consider Bowerman to have been the single most influential American coach in the area of training distance runners. Many other coaches and writers feel the same way.

While giving me an interview for an article, Bowerman described a drill he had learned from the previous Oregon coach, Bill Hayward. The drill is very simple, similar to high knees, except that instead of raising your knees high, you keep them low and move your feet as rapidly as you can: *Pop! Pop! Pop! Pop!* Your arms move equally fast in short arcs.

But that wasn't the only thing I learned. I couldn't help but take advantage of Bowerman's expertise. So I asked him, "What are the secrets of running fast—if that isn't too basic a question?"

"No, it's a good question," he said. "I did an article with somebody once

(continued on page 200)

FLEXIBILITY DRILLS THAT BUILD SPEED

To avoid sore muscles, you should always warm up before (by jogging and stretching) and cool down after doing any drills that are designed to add flexibility or speed to your runs. When starting a dynamic flexibility program, begin with only one or two drills, and gradually increase your capacity over a period of weeks and months. These drills are best done on your easy days, when you are running short and have more time to concentrate on nonspecific training activities.

They are also best conducted in warm weather, when you can utilize soft, smooth grass surfaces. Living in the Midwest, I used to consider flexibility drills as more of a summer activity. Then my wife Rose and I bought a second home in Ponte Vedra Beach, Florida, offering me new and different training options. The flat and firm Atlantic beach is perfect for most of these drills. I also recommend a rubberized track, where members of local high school teams often train. Obviously, any training regimen detailed in this or another book must be adapted to fit the realities of each runner's situation.

To do the drills, you need a straightaway 50 to 75 meters long, preferably grass or another soft surface. My grandson Kyle, a running coach, recommends two to four repetitions of each of the drills, in the following order.

1. **High knees.** Probably the simplest drill, high knees is little more than running in place while moving forward gradually. Lift your knees high and land on the balls of your feet. Point your toes, with all movement straight ahead. Your arms pump high in countermovement to your legs. Coach Sam Bell warns against doing high knees too fast, which may make it difficult to do the movements correctly.

2. **Fast feet.** The late Bill Bowerman described fast feet as one means of teaching form to sprinters. This drill resembles high knees, except instead of emphasizing knee lift, you concentrate on moving your feet rapidly, almost pitter-patter. Straight-ahead movement with pointed toes is equally important here.

3. **High heels.** This exercise is easier than the two previous ones, and can be used at this point partly to catch your breath. Runners new to flexibility drills should master this drill before attempting the

next two drills. Simply run in place like high knees, but kick your legs high in back instead of lifting your knees. Relax during this drill, and don't overemphasize speed.

4. **Skipping for height.** To skip, you must push off one foot and land on that same foot before bringing your lead foot down. It's like the first two jumps of track and field's triple jump (formerly called the more descriptive "hop, step, and jump"). Skipping involves a pause, like the syncopated beat in music. In skipping for height (as with high knees), emphasis is on high knee lift. During the pause, while suspended in midair, focus on getting your knee as high as possible.

5. **Skipping for distance.** This is the same as skipping for height, except the emphasis is on distance. Remember to keep all movement in a straight line. The two skipping drills require good flexibility, but they also promote flexibility. It could be said that the first three drills help warm you up for the skipping drills.

6. **Bounding.** This is an elongated running action in which you concentrate on lifting your knees and striding with your arms up. It will become running unless you focus on high knee lift. You also might compare this drill to the first stage of the triple jump, the hop. That is not an easy drill to master. I would recommend it only to advanced runners.

7. **Double leg hop.** As with bounding, this is not a drill for inexperienced runners. The movement is similar to that in drill 3, high heels. Stand in place and hop, kicking both heels in back. The distance covered is unimportant.

Once you master these speed-improvement drills and can do them without excessive fatigue or postworkout soreness, you can integrate them into different parts of your training week. Try them in the middle of your medium-distance workouts. I sometimes include several of the drills as part of my prerace warmup. High knees, high heels, and fast feet work well to loosen me up.

Also, don't ignore the stepping or standing variations of these drills. They may be more suitable for cold weather conditions or for those for whom too-vigorous drilling raises an unnecessary risk.

on the secrets of speed. It was published in *Sports Illustrated* in 1968. And basically I was telling what Hayward taught me. It's very elemental: A straight line is the shortest distance between two points. My line mechanics were so bad that my foot would fly out to the side. One of the things that Hayward had me do was lean up against a wall and watch my feet. I would bring my leg through like this to try to get the feel of my leg moving in a straight line. (Bowerman leaned against his fireplace and slowly rotated his leg to mimic a sprinter's stride.) One leg, then the other. I've done this with a lot of people, and it works."

"The second thing was reaction time," continues Bowerman. (He jogged in place, his feet pitter-pattering at a rapid pace.) "You stand like this and gradually speed up your legs. . . . The reaction of bouncing the feet rapidly, then bringing the knees up slowly, trying to keep everything straight ahead, picking up the rhythm—but you don't do it only with the legs. You have to use the arms, because that's the way you're wired. By gradually speeding up the arms, you speed up the legs. Then, use the sprint distances as merely a measure of testing; how much is this fellow improving? We did sprint drills three times a week. High knee, fast leg, and sprint 40 yards. Simple drills: everything straight ahead, reaction time, mechanics of running. If there's some bad habit, work on it. For every action, there's an equal and opposite reaction.

"That was what Hayward did for me. I never knew how fast I was. I couldn't beat anybody; I was the slowest man on the high school team. After Hayward was through with me, the only man I couldn't beat was our university sprinter, Paul Starr, who was third in the National AAU Championships."

"So you were able to improve the speed of your sprinters with these simple drills of Bill Hayward's," I asked.

"And what works for sprinters applies to other runners as well," Bowerman explained. "God determines how fast you're going to run; I can help only with the mechanics."

Bowerman's successor as track coach at Oregon, Bill Dellinger, later described the fast-foot drill in an article in *Runner's World* magazine: "The concept behind this is to see how fast you can make your feet move. Unlike the high-knees drill, you barely lift your knees at all. The emphasis is on quickness. Don't stride out. Simply move your feet as if you were running over hot coals. You're teaching your feet to react quickly."

TWO ADVANCED DRILLS

There are two additional flexibility drills that are worth mentioning. However, I don't necessarily recommend them for all (particularly older) runners, because of the stress they place on the joints. These drills are bounding and the double leg hop.

Bounding is an elongated running action in which you concentrate on lifting your knees and pumping with your arms up. This is not running. You bound. You hop from one leg to the other: left, right, left, right, getting as high off the ground as you can. Focus on your knee lift. Add this to your repertoire of flexibility drills only after you are well-practiced in the other drills and your leg muscles are sufficiently strong enough to perform what is admittedly a very vigorous exercise.

The double leg hop also is not a drill for inexperienced runners. The movement is similar to what is done in the high heels drill, except that in the double leg hop you stand in place and hop, kicking both heels in the back. The distance covered is unimportant. Add this to your routine last. (My son Kevin would use this final drill only when in top shape.) It's worth noting that I've already subtracted it from mine; at my age, it's too dynamic and my risk of injury is too high.

The late Edmund R. Burke, PhD, an exercise physiologist who worked with the US Cycling Team, warned that like any other type of training, bounding drills can lead to poor results if not used properly. "Symptoms of tendinitis and synovitis, particularly of the knee, can result from too much plyometric training," said Dr. Burke.

Drills that promote dynamic flexibility—whether called bounding or plyometrics or ballistic stretching—do have their obvious place in the training program of a high school cross-country team. Kids enjoy doing them and can show off with the drills during their warmups. The well-trained athletes on college teams, such as those at Indiana and Oregon, also benefit by adding bounding to their program. However, for distance runners some plyometric drill work is beneficial, but I don't recommend exercises that involve jumping on and off boxes and sideboards. The risk of injury may be too great for many high-mileage runners, especially those in the masters ranks, who aren't used to speed drills or have limited flexibility.

Nevertheless, I believe that any runner can benefit by eventually adding at least some of the drills covered in this chapter to his or her training regimen. Benson's experience at his running camps would suggest that this is so, since he has taught speed drills to many adult runners who have attended his camps. Just make sure to listen to your body.

CHAPTER EIGHTEEN

THE 15K

How to run your fastest time
at this unique distance

What I liked best about the Blueberry Stomp was the ceremonial stomping of blueberries. The 15K race was held each Labor Day in Plymouth, a small town just south of South Bend, Indiana. The race was part of that town's annual blueberry festival. Centerpiece for the long weekend festival was a parade on Monday, watched each year by an estimated 50,000 spectators, many of whom would arrive an hour or two early and position folding chairs on lawns to reserve their viewing spaces. The Blueberry Stomp began on Plymouth's main street immediately before the parade.

In an era when only the Boston Marathon attracted much attention, runners loved the fame this race brought them and the opportunity to experience the roar of the crowd. How often does someone who just started jogging get an opportunity to strut their stuff in front of 50,000 spectators, to become prologue for a huge celebratory parade?

Just before that moment, however, race founder Jeff Gangloff would appear with a bucket of blueberries and scatter them on the pavement in front of the waiting runners. This was part of the ritual. Jeff then would invite me, as the only semi-celebrity in the race, to stomp on the blueberries. And once the race began, all the other runners would stomp away, crossing the line until nothing remained of the blueberries except purple stains on the pavement.

What was there not to love about a road race with such a colorful beginning? I enjoyed the Stomp not only because of my role as primary stomper, but also because of the course; it was scenic and bucolic. I also liked it because the 15K distance is perhaps my favorite road race distance. The Stomp headed south through downtown, but quickly we reached the countryside, passing a cemetery, over a creek, cornstalks on either side of the road. The course was out-and-back with a loop in the middle. The last mile of the race was same as the first, meaning we finished on the parade route. Though relegated to a narrow corridor near the gutter, all runners thrilled to the incredible sights and sounds of cheering spectators and marching bands. Fifteen kilometers of running: my favorite distance.

BORN TO RUN THE 15K

Everybody has a favorite racing distance. Mine has always been 15 kilometers. (I also favored 10-mile races, just a bit longer than the 9.3-mile 15K.) There is a sound reason for my devotion to the 15K: I was born to run it. On the track, I did not have the speed to compete successfully at 1500 meters, the metric mile. On the roads, I did not have the endurance to beat the best in the marathon. But 15K: ah, that provided a perfect storm. Rivals, who might outkick me even in a 10K, often would see me fly past them in the final 3 miles of a 15K. I'm not entirely sure why. Maybe it was because the extra length of the race allowed me to fall into a rhythm that matched perfectly my stride length for 45 minutes, a time I was capable of when in my prime. Forty-five minutes: that is also a good length of time to be out running, no matter what your level of ability, no matter how many miles you might cover in that time. Ask me the best length of time, for instance, for a tempo run, and I will tell you 45 minutes.

I particularly remember the year when I ran the Stomp a few weekends after returning from the World Masters Championships in Toronto. After some of my best-ever months training, I had arrived at that championship track and field meet perfectly prepared, fine-tuned both mentally and physically. My feet had wings. I flew, winning the 3000 meter steeplechase in a time that still stands as the American age-group record 40 years later, the oldest on the books. I also placed third in the 10,000 meter cross-country race behind runners from England and New Zealand, among their country's best when younger.

Glory behind me, I arrived at the Stomp with nothing left to prove, with no fears of failure, with the knowledge that I was about to run another great race, no matter the competition. It mattered little that the fastest runners in the Stomp that day all were 10 to 20 years younger than me. I would stomp them after I stomped the blueberries. I started fast, and as we moved from town to countryside, I arrogantly attached myself to the shoulder of a friend, whose running resume included a 2:16 marathon, fast enough to gain entry into the Olympic Trials.

Somewhere after we strode past the 5K mark, I recall him looking at me over one shoulder. The look on his face said, "Are you still here?" He picked up the pace, and I stayed with him. We passed the 10K mark in a time faster than I ever had run that distance, either on the roads or on the track. By the time we returned to town, however, he had dropped me. But I still flew down the parade route in front of those 50,000 cheering spectators, few of them knowing that I had just run one of the fastest races in my life over one of my favorite distances. Finishing in second place, my name made no list of Blueberry Stomp winners. My time made no record books. I don't remember what happened to the trophy I won that day or if the Stomp even offered race T-shirts. No matter. The Blueberry Stomp that day lives in my memory, even if it does not live in the memory of anyone else.

What training do you need to do to run 15 kilometers (or its kissing cousin, 10 miles) and finish with a smile on your face? Yes, you need to train somewhat harder than you did using the 5K, 8K, and 10K programs already presented in this book. But you won't have to train that much harder, even though my 15K training programs feature an extra 2 weeks, 10 weeks total.

TWO MORE WEEKS

Those 2 extra weeks should help you easily make the jump from the 10K to the 15K. If you are a novice runner who has already begun to feel comfortable running a 10K, your training has put this longer distance within reach. The 15K Novice program offers the uptick in distance you need. Tuesday runs are somewhat longer, peaking at 5 miles. Midweek cross-training also is about the same, increasing from 30 to 45 minutes during the program's 10 weeks. Cycling, swimming, walking remain the best cross-training exercises, because they are aerobic. Thursday's mileage is less than Tuesday's mileage, recognizing the fact that you will have trained three consecutive days. Mondays and Fridays are rest days.

The key workout in the 15K program is the long run on Saturday, beginning with 2 miles in Week 1, peaking at 8 miles in Week 9, 1 week out from the race. You don't need to prove in advance that you can run 15K; save the extra 1.3 miles for the race itself. The step back in distance offers runners a psychological break. Thus in Week 4 and also in Week 7, you run slightly less than you might in a straight-line mileage progression. Have the exercise scientists offered any well-studied physiological reason for inserting this stepback week? Not really, but runners using my programs usually appreciate the opportunity for a brief break. Cross-training on Sundays—starting at 30 minutes and peaking at 60 minutes—offers a day of dynamic recovery. Here is my 15K training program for novice runners.

The 15K Novice

WEEK	MON	TUE	WED	THU	FRI	SAT	SUN
1	Rest	2 mile run	30 min cross	2 mile run	Rest	2 mile run	30 min cross
2	Rest	3 mile run	30 min cross	2 mile run	Rest	3 mile run	30 min cross
3	Rest	3 mile run	35 min cross	2 mile run	Rest	4 mile run	30 min cross
4	Rest	2 mile run	35 min cross	2 mile run	Rest	2 mile run	40 min cross
5	Rest	4 mile run	40 min cross	3 mile run	Rest	5 mile run	40 min cross
6	Rest	4 mile run	40 min cross	3 mile run	Rest	6 mile run	50 min cross
7	Rest	3 mile run	45 min cross	3 mile run	Rest	4 mile run	50 min cross
8	Rest	5 mile run	45 min cross	3 mile run	Rest	7 mile run	60 min cross
9	Rest	5 mile run	45 min cross	3 mile run	Rest	8 mile run	60 min cross
10	Rest	3 mile run	30 min cross	2 mile run	Rest	Rest	15K race

The intermediate program for 15K runners represents the next step upward. It also lasts 10 weeks, although the mileage on most days is somewhat higher than in the novice program. A bigger difference is the addition of a day of speedwork, midweek on Wednesdays.

Rest days remain the same: Mondays and Fridays. Take a full day off. If you do want to run a few miles on either of these days, I will not stand in your way. Keep the pace easy. Do not overtrain. Tuesday runs follow a pattern of 4 miles one week, 5 miles the next week, then 6 miles on the final week of a 3-week cycle. What's the purpose of this 4-5-6 pattern? No purpose other than to offer you some variety in your training and perhaps a change of pace depending on how far you go on a given day. Midweek is an alternating blend of interval workouts and timed tempo runs that begin at 30 minutes and reach 45 minutes at the maximum. Don't worry too much about matching precisely the time prescription, including on Sundays with their 60-minute maximum.

The key to the program, and the most important day that will benefit your progression from novice to intermediate runner, is Wednesday, the speedwork day. For variety, the program offers interval training at the track on odd weeks and tempo runs on the roads (or in the woods) on even weeks. Can you do interval workouts on the roads or do tempo runs on a track? I'll let you make that decision. Where you do any one workout is much less important than how you do that workout. Don't kill yourself doing a Wednesday workout, but you should finish feeling pleasantly fatigued, also knowing that the mileage on Thursday, the next day, is slightly less.

Long runs on Saturdays increase from 6 miles to 10 miles at the end of Week 9, which is one week out from your 15K. Note that this Week 9 run is actually slightly longer than your race distance. As an intermediate runner, whether or not you can finish 15K in style and speed should not worry you. Note the addition of a test race halfway through the program at the end of Week 5. I suggest a 10K race, but it could be any distance between 5K and 10K, and if there is a fun race on a slightly different weekend, don't be afraid to modify the schedule. Here then is my 15K training program for intermediate runners.

The 15K Intermediate

WEEK	MON	TUE	WED	THU	FRI	SAT	SUN
1	Rest	4 mile run	4 × 800 5K pace	2 mile run	Rest	6 mile run	60 min cross
2	Rest	5 mile run	30 min tempo	3 mile run	Rest	7 mile run	60 min cross
3	Rest	6 mile run	5 × 800 5K pace	4 mile run	Rest	8 mile run	60 min cross
4	Rest	4 mile run	35 min tempo	2 mile run	Rest	4 mile run	60 min cross
5	Rest	5 mile run	6 × 800 5K pace	3 mile run	Rest	Rest	10K test
6	Rest	6 mile run	40 min tempo	4 mile run	Rest	8 mile run	60 min cross
7	Rest	4 mile run	7 × 800 5K pace	2 mile run	Rest	4 mile run	60 min cross
8	Rest	5 mile run	45 min tempo	3 mile run	Rest	9 mile run	60 min cross
9	Rest	6 mile run	8 × 800 5K pace	4 mile run	Rest	10 mile run	60 min cross
10	Rest	4 mile run	30 min tempo	3 mile run	1-2 mile run	Rest	15K race

We come now to the advanced program for runners committed to my favorite distance, the 15K. While I also offer programs that last longer (12 weeks for the half marathon, 18 weeks for the full) and have more mileage, both daily and weekly, I'm not certain they necessarily are more difficult than the 15K Advanced program I provide here. Maybe I should not even suggest that one program is more difficult than another. Depending on your own natural ability, depending on how much previous training you might have done during a short or long running career, any program might be considered either hard or easy. Having said that, this may be the most difficult program in this book, and its blend of speed and endurance is designed to help you run fast.

I know the type of runner who might be attracted to this program. You don't like to take a day off. "Rest" is a word that not all advanced runners understand, sometimes to their detriment. As an advanced runner, you want to run seven days a week, and I'm going to let you do just that. You might have done some hard training over the weekend, but an easy 3-miler on Mondays should not be a problem for someone at this level. One criticism I sometimes hear from experienced runners is that many of my programs are low in mileage. My response is that, depending on your ability, you can always add mileage, either in small doses, like adding a mile or two to a pre-scribed 3-mile run, or doing a second workout. In all of my advanced pro-grams I focus more on quality than quantity. If you can handle more quantity (i.e., more miles), be my guest, but don't add so many miles to this program so that quality suffers.

I would count tempo runs as quality runs. In the 15K Advanced program they are on Tuesdays, the length of each run increasing from 30 to 45 min-utes. Start easy, accelerate to a faster pace in the middle, hold it, and finish easy. Each runner needs to determine how hard to run this workout. Keep in mind that if you run too hard on Tuesdays, you may struggle doing the equally hard workouts on Wednesdays—interval training on the track. Thursdays are easy runs. If you want to include strength training as part of your workout week, then Mondays and Thursdays would be the best days. Run first, then head to the gym. You will find that sequence easier than running after a gym workout, since lifting tightens the muscles. An easy run before lifting should loosen the muscles.

Friday is an option day: run or rest. The toughest workouts come on the weekends: pace runs on Saturdays, long runs on Sundays. By "pace" I mean the pace at which you hope to run in your 15K race. "Goal pace" is another way to state this. Learning to run a perfect pace will help you to become a faster runner. You want to avoid those last-mile slowdowns that come because you went out too fast in the early miles. The long runs begin at 5 miles and end at 13 miles, well over your race distance. But as an advanced runner, you should have no trouble running this far. No cross-training in this program, recognizing the fact that most advanced runners want to run, want only to run, and don't want to spend time on other activities. If you don't fit that pattern and would like to cross-train, Mondays or Thursdays might be the best days on which to do so. Here then is my training program for advanced 15K runners.

The 15K Advanced

WEEK	MON	TUE	WED	THU	FRI	SAT	SUN
1	3 mile run	30 min tempo run	6 × 400 mile pace	3 mile run	Rest or 3 mile run	3 mile pace	5 mile run
2	3 mile run	35 min tempo run	3 × 800 5K pace	4 mile run	Rest or 3 mile run	4 mile pace	6 mile run
3	3 mile run	40 min tempo run	7 × 400 mile pace	5 mile run	Rest or 3 mile run	5 mile pace	7 mile run
4	3 mile run	30 min tempo run	4 × 800 5K pace	3 mile run	Rest or 3 mile run	Rest	**5K race**
5	3 mile run	40 min tempo run	8 × 400 mile pace	4 mile run	Rest or 3 mile run	4 mile pace	9 mile run
6	3 mile run	45 min tempo run	5 × 800 5K pace	5 mile run	Rest or 3 mile run	5 mile pace	10 mile run
7	3 mile run	30 min tempo run	9 × 400 mile pace	3 mile run	Rest or 3 mile run	Rest	**10K race**
8	3 mile run	40 min tempo run	6 × 800 5K pace	4 mile run	Rest or 3 mile run	5 mile pace	12 mile run
9	3 mile run	45 min tempo run	10 × 400 mile pace	5 mile run	Rest or 3 mile run	6 mile pace	13 mile run
10	3 mile run	30 min tempo run	3 × 800 5K pace	2 mile run	1-2 mile run	Rest	**15K race**

CHAPTER NINETEEN

HIT THE HILLS
Climb your way to the top

The University of Oregon's Bill Bowerman was known for his bluntness. I once quizzed him about whether training on hills could make you a better runner. "When they start putting hills on tracks," he replied gruffly, "I'll have my athletes run hills in practice."

It was a classic remark from a classic coach. Specificity of exercise is important for any sport, which is one reason why I don't over-prescribe either cross-training or strength training. Yet Arthur Lydiard, the New Zealand coach whom Bowerman admitted using as a source for many training ideas, strongly recommended hill training for those wanting to improve their speed on track or road.

Exercise physiologist Dean Brittenham also believes that one way runners get stronger (thus faster) is to run up an incline. "Most good training programs have one common philosophy—some type of resistance running," he says. "And the best way to achieve that is with hills."

Many runners realize this and incorporate hill training into their regular workout routines. Cindy Jackson Knull, 46, a stay-at-home mom from Tulsa, Oklahoma, lives in a very hilly area. "It's part of my regular training runs, therefore I do not do hill repeats. I'm ready for hills at any time in a race as a result."

Jessica Ibsen, 34, a marketing consultant from Slidell, Louisiana, states, "In southern Louisiana, hills are nonexistent. I actually drive about 30 minutes to a place in Mississippi so I can run a 7.5 mile loop of hills. My friend and I did that for a month before a race in hilly Kentucky to prepare us for the change in terrain. We would have been in some real trouble had we not had those weekly hill sessions."

Jessie Bigger, 30, an athletic trainer from Helotes, Texas, lives on the fringe of the hill country in San Antonio. "There is no way to avoid hills here. Last year I trained for my first full marathon, choosing to run my weekly runs in our neighborhood pushing my then 1-year-old son. I effectively dropped from 10-minute miles at the start of training to 8:30-minute miles at the end. I fully believe the hills made me stronger and faster."

I have a similar situation, living just over the crest of a hill that rises about 75 feet above the shores of Lake Michigan. The road in front of my house is relatively flat to the west, sloping slightly downward. To the east, however, the road dips more precipitously, losing most of its above-lake altitude within several hundred yards before starting to level off. So right out my front door, I have a nearly one-quarter-mile hill that's perfect for resistance training.

When I run east on Lakeshore Drive, I must begin downhill, which can be painful on days when I am tight from the previous day's hard workout. Returning, I must cope with this hill in the closing minute of my run.

The "Higdon Hill" was a pivotal part of the 15K course used for the Michigan City Run, a major local race. Runners headed down the hill midway through the fourth mile, made a U-turn farther down the road, and came back up it just before the 6-mile mark. The hill therefore became the break point where many races were either won or lost.

When Bill Rodgers ran Michigan City in 1978, I pointed out to him that the hill steepens just before the crest. Once over the top, however, he could use the quick drop and the gentle decline that follows over the next half-mile to gain momentum for a long surge to the finish. And that's where Rodgers left the other competitors in the race.

LEARNING TO LOVE HILLS

Let's talk about hills. Uphills and downhills. Big hills and small hills. Hills as both aid and deterrent to performance. Hills in training and hills in races. Hills as both a cause and a preventive of injuries. How to run them and how to avoid them. What to do when you don't have them, yet you still have to race on a hilly course. Hills to build strength and hills to build speed. Hills to build courage and hills to discourage. Are they an essential training tool or a gimmick dreamed up by some New Zealand coach out to prove to joggers that they'll never make it as serious racers?

The coach was Arthur Lydiard, and he outlined hill running in his books and numerous lectures as an essential ingredient of his three-step training buildup.

1. Endurance training

2. Hill training

3. Speedwork

Lydiard did not discover hill training, however, any more than Zebulon Montgomery Pike discovered the mountain peak bearing his name. The Native Americans arrived at the peak before Pike, and Percy Cerutty was using hills before Lydiard to train Australian runners such as Herb Elliott, 1500-meter champion at the 1960 Olympics in Rome. Cerutty used to send Elliott sprinting up sand dunes near his training center at Portsea. Even before Cerutty, there were other coaches and runners who advocated hill running to build stamina, although Cerutty may have been the only coach to claim that running at full pace up a hill could bring "relief from constipation."

Lydiard made no such claims. He was less a discoverer of hill training than one who developed a systemized program that utilized hills as a key training ingredient. Lydiard's runners, including Olympic champions Murray Halberg and Peter Snell, did not merely run hills, they trained on them at specific points in their season to prepare for specific races.

Lydiard's hill workouts had a pattern. His athletes would run a 5-mile warmup, then run up a half-mile hill, run one-quarter mile fast on top, run hard downhill, and run one-quarter mile of quick fartlek at the bottom. They'd do six or eight of these hill loops, followed by a 2-mile cooldown. This was hardly the sort of workout schedule you would suggest to a beginner, but after Lydiard's runners started to win at the Olympics, track fans began to ask, what is it that they are doing differently? The answer was they were running hills.

Although Lydiard's endorsement was unequivocal, the research is inconclusive. Studies related to the specificity of exercise suggest that if you plan to race on hills, you need to train on hills. But whether such training also makes you a better runner on the flats and on the track is difficult to measure in the laboratory. (Apparently, Bowerman's reasoning for not recommending hill training to track athletes was well founded.) But Lydiard believed that running up and down

If you plan to race on hills, you need to train on hills.

hills can make you a faster runner— and the achievements of his athletes would seem to support him.

ADVOCATES AND SKEPTICS

Research by exercise physiologist Jack Daniels, PhD, determined that the addition of hill running does indeed increase the intensity of a training program. A runner's energy cost, he found, increases by 12 percent when running up a 1-degree slope, but only 7 percent of the energy returns when coming down that same slope.

Jack H. Wilmore, PhD, supervised a project by graduate students Doug Allen and Beau Freund while at the University of Arizona. They trained two groups of runners, one on the flats, the other running a gradual stadium ramp. At the end of the study, they found no difference between the two groups, at least not in the changes of their VO_2 max. "That tells you something," says Dr. Wilmore, "although maybe athletes don't want to hear it." Dr. Wilmore and his team did not measure performance by testing the runners on a track or in races, so it is possible that hill training might have some important mental benefits that are not easily measurable, convincing runners they are tougher.

Leslie Stapp, 52, a psychotherapist from Whittier, California, uses hills as a substitute for track work. She says: "Give me miles of crazy hills out on a woodsy trail over the track any day. I know I probably should track train too, but I will seek out hills and even drive to them, using every excuse in the book to avoid the track."

David L. Costill, PhD, maintains that, theoretically, hill training should improve speed. "In order to have good speed," he says, "you must create force through the thigh and hamstring muscles, and hill work develops both." But Dr. Costill admitted to not having researched the subject.

"Hill training is another form of resistance," claims E. C. Frederick, PhD. "All training boils down to cleverly increasing the amount of resistance that your body can adapt to. So, running uphill is one way of tricking the body. But there is no magic to hill training, no special adaptation that you can't get somewhere else."

Bob Glover, coauthor of *The Runner's Handbook* and head of the New York Road Runners Club's coaching program, believes that if you plan to race on hills, you need to train on hills. He offers several reasons, however, why even runners racing on flat courses should consider training on hills.

- Uphill intervals can be used to improve your form. You must concentrate on form to get up the hill.

- Downhill runs can teach relaxation and improve leg speed and stride.

- Hill running is "speedwork in disguise." It can be used in place of track workouts to improve your anaerobic efficiency.

- Hills strengthen your legs, especially your quads, lessening the possibility of knee injury.

- Your mental ability to handle hills in races improves.

Glover adds, "If you live in the flatlands, be creative. Highway ramps or parking garages are possibilities, although they may pose obvious safety problems."

ELITE ADVICE ON HILLS

Whether to build strength or to condition themselves for hilly races, most top runners use hills in their training. Bill Rodgers, who in his prime had an excellent reputation as a hill runner (particularly on the descent), was among them. He once told me, "First, as an uphill runner, I'm weak. I've tried to do more hill repeats to compensate for this. Downhill, my success may be just from the way I land, my lightness. But even in high school, my coach emphasized pushing over the hill and not running as hard going up.

"I don't practice downhill running. The only time I would run hills was before Boston. I started to do more uphill training when I saw how well Randy Thomas and Greg Meyer ran on the uphills."

Rodgers used to train on none other than the infamous Heartbreak Hill, the fourth of the Newton hills that comes near the 21-mile mark on the course of the Boston Marathon. Although Heartbreak Hill is not particularly steep, it is about 600 yards long and is the make or break point for many marathoners. Rodgers would run on the grass parkway beside the road, doing 6 to 10 repeats in 1:35. Between uphill bursts, he would jog back down, letting the grass cushion the impact of the downhill (an important step in injury prevention). "I see a lot of other runners training on Heartbreak," says Rodgers, "particularly before Boston."

When Olympic gold medalist Joan Benoit Samuelson coached at Boston University, she often took her team there. "The girls on the team enjoyed it," recalls Samuelson. They would do five to eight repeats. Other times, they ran Summit Avenue Hill, several miles from Heartbreak but not on the marathon course. Samuelson notes that it usually took her team 2 to 3 days to recover after a workout on Summit.

"Living in Boston back then, I didn't get onto hills that often," she commented on the training that led her to an Olympic marathon victory in 1984. "During the course of a run, if I came to a hill, I would really charge it." Now living in her native state of Maine, Samuelson has more access to hilly running areas.

Herb Lindsay, formerly a number one–ranked road runner, lived in

Boulder, Colorado, where the Flatiron Mountains rise several thousand feet above the city. Large canyons feature numerous uphill and downhill trails for training. Lindsay felt that the rolling plains before the Colorado Front Range also offered an opportunity for specific hill training, although he preferred to call it incline training.

"At altitude, one of the negative factors is that you can't get the quality of speed training you can at sea level," Lindsay explains. "You're limited by the thin air, but you can compensate by running on a gentle descent. With gravity pushing you along, you can run as fast (that is, with the same leg speed) as you can at sea level. I did train on uphills, but I probably used downhills with more planning."

ADVICE FOR FLATLANDERS

One strong believer in hill training is former American 5000-meter record holder Marty Liquori. This may seem strange when you consider that Liquori lives in Gainesville, Florida, which is as flat as one of coach Bowerman's tracks. As a substitute for hills, Liquori ran the stadium steps at the University of Florida. He says, "My feeling is that if Arthur Lydiard had a stadium in Auckland like we have in Gainesville, he would promote stadium running. Florida's stadium seats 70,000 people and has three levels of incline that get progressively steeper; it takes 35 seconds to reach the top, and nobody can run up it more than about eight times."

Liquori would train there once or twice a week before the track season. In between "uphills," he sometimes would run an easy 4 × 400 on the track to loosen up, then go back up the stadium. "At the end, you're totally rigged," he recalls.

Liquori's "stadiums uphills" can be compared with Lydiard's half-mile hills, coming as they did during a specific segment of his training year. Liquori ran the stadium in a transition period between distance running and track work. "When you run a lot of distance, your stride shortens," says Liquori. "Your leg muscles are not extending, so they become fairly weak. You go to a hill phase to make a transition, to force you to open up your stride by bounding up hills. You exaggerate knee lift and arm swing, push off with the toes and calves. This strengthens your quadriceps and buttocks muscles before going back onto the track. It's right out of the Lydiard book."

Another important factor, believes Liquori, is that somebody who has limited time for training can fatigue the muscles more rapidly on hills than on the flats. "When I was traveling and knew I had only a half-hour to work out," he says, "I'd look for a hill. I could get more exhausted than doing a 90-minute run."

In a situation where you have neither mountains nor a stadium nearby, yet you face scheduled races on hilly courses, you may need to try another training modification. Two-time Olympian Fred Wilt said, "If you are not going to run uphill in training, you have to do a lot of running where you go at one pace, then cut loose for 50 yards. The energy requirements for going uphill are so much greater than on the flats, you have to get used to higher energy expenditures in a race."

Still another option is to use a treadmill with an adjustable incline. Many runners belong to health clubs or gyms that have treadmills and other exercise machines that can be used to develop the same muscles.

You don't need to be a world class runner to benefit from hill training. Pam Triest-Hallahan, 55, a math teacher from Nashua, New Hampshire, lives at the top of a very hilly neighborhood. "I love to run up the big hills," she admits. "I often find that 'hilly' race courses just have a bump or two compared to my usual routes."

Nancy Lehr, 52, a pharmacist from Lawton, Oklahoma, describes her favorite course of 4 or 5 miles used for group runs. "Part of that route is also in our half marathon," says Lehr. "Sometimes our workouts are not very fun, but we always call it 'thrills on the hills.'"

Jack Duysen, 56, a contractor from Omaha, Nebraska, admits to having a love/hate relationship with hills. "I live in a very hilly neighborhood, so I run hills almost every day. I dread hill repeats, but I do them because in races I pass a lot of people who can't attack hills."

You don't need to be a world class runner to benefit from hill training.

USING HILLS TO BUILD MUSCLE

Fellow coach and running guru Jeff Galloway wrote in an article in *Runner's World* magazine, "Many coaches and strength experts believe hills provide better strength for running than weights or machines. Pushing up the incline builds the lower leg muscles. With power there, you can develop a more efficient push-off, better running posture, and more strength in your legs.

"Weight lifting strengthens those same muscles, but it won't train them for the demands of running. The large and small muscles in the legs must work together perfectly to produce a smooth stride. Hill running builds strength and coordination at the same time."

When Ron Gunn coached distance runners at Southwestern Michigan College in Dowagiac, he often used a 200-meter sloping fairway on a golf course near the campus. There, he had his team do circuit sprinting on the grass following a fast run of 5 to 7 miles. He called the circuit Scando-loops after the Scandinavians.

Here's how Gunn defined the workout. "Go at a faster-than-race pace up the hill, then do a relaxing jog around the top. Run easily the first 75 meters of the downhill that is steep; then when the drop begins to level out, relax and lift up on the balls of your feet, arms vertical, and sprint down the hill. It's what we call going into fifth gear. Get back down to the bottom, then jog some more, sprint again at the bottom, jog some more, go up again. Do about six of those. It develops speed and strength, and it also teaches you to run a hill properly."

Another Gunn circuit on an old country road featured a hill with three levels, where his runners alternated fast and slow running according to the pitch of the hill. Gunn had his squad run hills twice a week for as many as 8 weeks prior to a major competition. Sometimes, the hills served as just one part of a structured program, other times, they made up the entire workout. He says, "Hills also are good for getting into condition quickly without the risk of injury. You don't have to do a lot of running to obtain a quality workout. You don't need as many repetitions."

Liquori adds, "With the caliber of runners we have today, they can't get tired doing interval work on a track. You could take a workout like 20 quarters in 55 seconds, and today's runners just might be able to do it. But before they finish, an Achilles tendon would flare up, or ligaments would give way. Running hills permits you to do more by doing less. When you get to the point where everybody runs 120 miles a week at a 5:30 pace, you have to find other ways to generate more stress. Hills may be the wave of the future."

One warning, however: Running hills strains the muscles, tendons, and ligaments of your feet, particularly the bottoms of your feet, because in running up an incline you push off from the ball of your foot. This strains the plantar fascia. You'll feel sharp pain on the heel (where the fascia connects) if you get this injury. It feels like a heel bruise, but is not. San Leandro, California, podiatrist Steven Subotnick, DPM, says that plantar fasciitis is a common injury in his area because runners do a lot of their training on hilly courses. If you plan to add hills to your training program, introduce them gradually. Think like a beginner. By moving slowly into hill training, you will decrease your risk of injury.

RUN TO THE TOP

Obviously, elite runners turn to hills to add an intensity to their workouts they just can't get anywhere else. But what about midpack runners? Coach Gunn has trained just such people in classes at his community college: men and women, young and old, with little background as competitive athletes. "They do circuits on the same hills," he says, "only involving different techniques. As with our college students, I'll have them do some kind of tempo run; then they'll end up in the latter stage of the workout doing hills. They'll start with three to four and build up to seven or eight, running faster than race pace, then turn around and jog down. They don't do the other phases.

"We run on golf courses or forest trails. We've gotten off hard roads now. It's pretty difficult to injure an athlete running up a hill. The time you have to be careful is coming down."

At the Nike Sport Research Lab, Tom Clark studied the impact shock of running up and down hills. Ten well-trained runners ran at various grades, from 6 percent uphill to 8 percent downhill, at a 7-minute-mile pace. At the steepest uphill grade, the shock was only 85 percent of that experienced running on level ground. The steepest downhill grade resulted in 40 percent more leg shock—an increased risk of injury.

It may be, then, that hill training—particularly intensive training—and running fast downhill should be reserved for days when you are well-rested and at a point during your workout where you are relaxed from a good warmup but not yet excessively fatigued. "You're more likely to injure yourself when you're tired," says Lindsay of his incline training.

Of course, what goes up must come down—or does it? Liquori claimed one trick he learned from world-class New Zealanders Rod Dixon and John Walker was to not run downhill. "Instead of 4-minute intervals on a track, they would go 10 minutes up a steep hill and get a ride back down," Liquori explains. That suggests the ultimate athletic perk: a driver waiting for you at the top of a mountain. Even without that, most runners who attempt hill training will find that it makes them better runners.

DEVELOP HILL TECHNIQUE

Once you agree that training on hills can make you a faster runner, you should be ready to develop a hill running technique. One summer, I taught at the Green Mountain Running Camp in northern Vermont. Each morning from our hilltop campus at Lyndon State College, I looked out over a rolling landscape. Fog settled in the valleys; hills above touched the sky. I wanted to run those hills forever.

But as I discovered from observing the runners at the camp, not everybody knows how to run hills—up or down. Their main form fault was not knowing how to lean. They leaned into the hill going up; they leaned backward going down. Actually, they should have been doing the opposite.

Uphills

Let's focus first on uphills, which trouble runners most. Runners can learn about hill running technique from skiers and cyclists. Going uphill,

Training on hills can make you a stronger runner.

a cross-country skier looks toward the top of the slope. Raising his gaze causes a slight shift backward in weight, anchoring each ski plant enough to avoid slipping. If the skier leans forward, the skis lose traction. At the end of cross-country ski races, I constantly have to fight the tendency to slump forward from fatigue, which causes my skis to slide backward.

The same is true in cycling. My first time on a mountain bike, I also learned quickly to sit back in the saddle going up the trail. When I did otherwise, my wheels spun. For best bike traction, you keep weight over the power (rear) wheel. The same is true for running: Learn to lean back when going uphill. Focusing on the top with your eyes will get you to the top.

Also, change your tempo when starting uphill. Just as a cyclist downshifts to accommodate the grade, runners need to change gears by shortening and quickening stride. But don't push too hard uphill; otherwise, you won't have enough stamina to run fast downhill.

Downhills

Running downhill takes another skill and a different attitude. In the closing miles of the Boston Marathon, people lining Commonwealth Avenue encourage runners by shouting: "It's downhill all the way!" Actually, most runners find it more difficult running down than up due to the immense impact. Uphill, you can survive on guts; downhill requires skill and practiced techniques.

I learned about downhill running from Kenny Moore, the 1968 and 1972 Olympic marathoner who writes for *Sports Illustrated*. During the course of researching hill running for a two-part article that appeared in *Runner's World* magazine, I was told by several runners that Moore was their downhill running guru. I contacted him and I discovered that he came out strong in favor of leaning forward while going down the hill, not holding back. Kenny Moore said: "Primary, I think, is raw smugness, preferably born of experience, which will let one bolt freewheeling down a slope without any fear of falling. That fear, I'm sure, works against the kind of relaxation necessary. It takes, at first anyway, a bit of nerve to lean forward so the torso is perpendicular to the surface of the hill, and to run with the same action and footplant one would use on the level. The idea, of course, is to let gravity do all the work, and that can't happen if you're clunking down on your heels or shooting the soles of your feet along the pavement."

Moore continued to say that downhill running takes practice as well, to condition the thighs to the intense pounding and to get the legs used to the much higher rates of stride. The main problem in downhill running, as Moore clearly understood, is attitude. Not mental attitude, but the way the astronauts use that term to describe positioning a space capsule. The right attitude for downhill runners is leaning forward. Just as you can learn from skiers and cyclists going uphill by leaning backward and shifting gears, you also can learn from these other athletes about running the downhills.

Going downhill, a skier keeps weight evenly distributed on his skis, but tilts forward from the waist into a tuck position to minimize wind drag. A cyclist does the same thing, tucking down on the handlebars to lower the body (and lessen resistance) as much as possible. As a runner, you need not worry as much about wind drag, but you also should tilt forward to let the hill carry you down. Not only will you go faster, but you minimize pounding by getting off your heels. Braking slows you and wastes the effort you just invested in running uphill.

Here's where attitude comes in: You want to tilt forward, not merely lean. The tilt begins at the pelvis and is ever so slight. To master this pelvic tilt, you need practice. Find a long downhill—not too steep—and experiment with different tilts as you run, seeing what angle changes do to both your speed and comfort.

Finally, know the courses where you plan to race. In preparing for the Boston Marathon, I always advise runners to practice downhill running as well as uphill running. The four Newton hills—including famous Heartbreak Hill—get a lot of publicity, but the course is overall more downhill than up with a drop of roughly 450 feet from the start in suburban Hopkinton to the finish on Boylston Street in downtown Boston.

Some of the Boston drop—such as that in the first mile—is noticeable, but other downhills are so subtle that you barely notice them. This is particularly true in the last 5 miles, which is where tired runners have the most difficulty coping with the downward slant. And it's where they do the most damage to their leg muscles because they no longer have the strength to maintain a forward-leaning position on the downhills, as recommended by Moore. They lose form and begin pounding. As a result, they spend the week after the race walking very stiff-legged.

One way to avoid at least some of the muscle damage that occurs is to train for the downhills. In running repeats on the hill in front of my house before Boston, I usually would run one downhill repeat for each two uphill repeats. There is a danger, however, in overdoing downhill training because of an increased risk of injury from the impact.

Nevertheless, training on hills can make you a stronger runner. And when it comes to running fast, strength equals speed—as we will discuss further in the next chapter.

CHAPTER TWENTY

STRENGTH TRAINING

*Lifting weight is no longer an
outlier activity for runners*

When the first running boom was getting started, beginning in the 1970s and continuing into the 1980s and 1990s, if I suggested to runners that they include some strength training in their workout routines, I got pushback. It was a tough sell. Runners just wanted to run. They enjoyed heading out the door and running the roads, or through the woods. Running was fun. Hanging out in a gym and pumping iron did not seem to be fun. This particularly appeared to be the mindset of the increasing number of women who were attracted to the sport of running.

Times have changed. Now the gym with all its glitzy machines has become easily accessible to both men and women. Strength training has become fun. The new breed of runner more often recognizes the advantage of having a well-balanced body. They hope that a little lifting will improve their general health, even if it might not help them run faster. The mindset of women also has changed. They no longer feel intimidated walking into a weight room that once was the sole province of muscle-bound men. And the guys now have become accustomed to having a gal lifting at the next bench.

Kim Dobson strength trains at home and in the gym: "My legs and body are much stronger because of the training. An added benefit is the inspiration and encouragement from others at the gym."

The most successful runners—those dominating the front of the race both in major marathons and local 5K races—tend to be skinny individuals with minimal body mass. "Running develops the lower body, but does little for the upper body," admits coach Tom Brunick. "The arm-swinging we do to counterbalance leg motion offers some development, but not much." There's also a question as to exactly how much benefit runners actually get from all the weightlifting and cross-training they might do for supplemental exercise. Will strength training help you run faster, or is it simply one more gimmick to sell exercise equipment and health club memberships?

Among those favoring strength training is Caitlin Alvaro, 29, a swimming instructor from Adelaide, Australia. Adding gym workouts to her regular running routine, Alvaro says, helped drop her 5K time by nearly 2 minutes: "I'm 100 percent convinced it has helped my speed."

Amber Hadigan, 41, a writer from Hyde Park, New York, does not go to a gym to strength train, preferring to use light weights at home and exercises tied to her body weight: "I have improved greatly by strengthening my core and back muscles. When my core is stronger, I can run longer."

Andrew Richter, 42, an editor from Cliffwood Beach, New Jersey, suggests another benefit. For him, weight lifting seems to equal weight

Will strength training help you run faster?

loss: "Since I got more serious about strength training, I've shaved off pounds I thought never would go away. I look the best I ever have, and my running has improved, too."

While some runners find that weight lifting or other forms of strength training do make a difference, many researchers concede that there is little conclusive evidence. The benefits are not easy to document, either on the track or in an exercise lab. It depends partly on your running event, partly on your ability, partly on how much you run. Most scientists concede that documented studies fail to demonstrate any benefit of weight lifting for young, male, elite runners—although they may for individuals in other categories. Studies at the University of Massachusetts in Amherst, for example, have shown strength gains of 10 to 15 percent among older runners who add weight training to their schedules. But Daniel Becque, PhD, who conducted the study, admits strength may be more important for sprinters than for distance runners. "For Olympic champion Haile Gebrselassie to suddenly start pumping iron would be fruitless," says Dr. Becque.

I've discussed the subject on several occasions with David L. Costill, PhD. He claims that strength training makes you a better weight lifter, but not necessarily a better runner. The reason is specificity of exercise. To run fast, you need to run fast. "There's no raw, objective data," he says, "that proves you will run faster if you weight train."

DOES STRENGTH TRAINING WORK?

Still, weight training does have its share of running advocates. Lawrence E. Armstrong, PhD, a former colleague of Dr. Costill, believes that power training can help improve your stride length—one element that separates fast runners from slow ones. While at Ball State, Dr. Armstrong collaborated with Dr. Costill on a study that attempted to measure the difference between sprinters and distance runners.

The sprinters were more muscular; the distance runners were more lean. Dr. Costill and Dr. Armstrong filmed the athletes during a maximum sprint. They noted that at maximum speed, the sprinters and distance runners had identical body angles: straight up. But they also found a revealing difference—stride lengths. At maximum velocity, the sprinters' stride lengths were longer than the distance runners', although stride frequencies were the same. Apparently, a longer stride is what permitted the sprinters to run faster for shorter distances. It gave them a special "kick."

"Because stride length, and not stride frequency, is paramount to speed production," Dr. Armstrong summarized in his report, "training should focus on the muscles which produce a long, powerful stride, namely the muscles of the hip, thigh, and lower leg." He noted that speedwork develops those muscles. He felt that the study supported those coaches who recommend power drills, such as uphill training and bounding, to improve leg strength, which consequently lengthens the stride. But he also suggested that weight lifting might add an "extra edge" and help to stabilize joints by strengthening the surrounding musculature.

Ask ordinary runners (not just sprinters or elite athletes) whether they can improve by adding strength training to their workout routine, and the answer is an unqualified "yes." I asked my running friends on Facebook to share their lifting experiences. The response was rapid, and positive.

Jen Barry, 33, a marketing manager from Austin, Texas, did not do any lifting before her first two marathons, because she did not understand the importance of strength training. "I finished," she says, "but not as well as I had hoped." Before her third marathon, Barry added one extra day of lifting to her regular training routine and knocked 20 minutes off her PR.

But, time out! Sounds like a great endorsement for strength training, but cause and effect may be difficult to prove. Exercise scientists do not always smile on anecdotal information. Having run two previous marathons—the learning experience, the build-up of miles—may have been more important to the 20-minute improvement than a single extra day of lifting.

James Jenkins, 41, a music instructor from Jackson, Mississippi, believes that in addition to the obvious benefits of strength training, there is a psychological benefit as well: "It lets you accomplish something rather challenging after having run for the day, and I like accomplishing things. It gives you another activity."

Despite the inconclusive scientific data, it is hard to ignore the positive benefits runners consistently report from strength training. The question that many runners, often those new to the gym, might ask is: "How do you do it?"

To increase the power output of the hip flexors, hip extensors, knee extensors, and ankle extensors, Dr. Armstrong recommends half squats, heel raises, and hip extensions. He warns that the transition to power training should be gradual to avoid ligament, muscle, or tendon damage.

Here are some weight-training exercises that can strengthen those parts of the body. For best results, lift 50 to 60 percent of the maximum weight you can lift in a set of 12 repetitions.

Half squats. Stand with your feet shoulder-width apart (or wider), with the weight of a barbell resting across your shoulders and behind your neck.

Bend your knees and lower your body until the tops of your thighs are parallel to the floor. Dr. Armstrong recommends that the descent be constant, slow, and controlled. The barbell should remain stable—that is, with very little movement forward or rearward. After reaching the bottom position, begin your ascent, keeping the movement constant but rapid. Complete the movement with a forward hip roll. (Deep squats are not recommended because of an increased risk of injury.) This exercise strengthens four muscles: the quadriceps, hamstrings, gluteals, and erector spinae.

Heel raises. Stand with your feet shoulder-width apart, a barbell resting on your shoulders behind your neck. Use a support block one-half to 1 inch high. Stand with the balls of your feet on the block and your heels on the ground, but otherwise in the same position as for the first exercise. Raise your heels off the ground so that all of your weight is forward, on your toes. Your movement should be deliberate and controlled. Return to the starting position and repeat. Even without weights, this is a good stretching exercise. This exercise strengthens the gastrocnemius and soleus, the main muscles of the lower leg.

Hip extensions. This exercise is best performed using an exercise machine that features cables and pulleys, with a brace on the end of the cable in which you can position your calf. Stand straight, facing the wall or the machine, and hold on to the machine for support. Your legs should be shoulder-width apart. Move the braced leg back to a 45-degree angle. Bend your support leg if necessary, but keep your braced leg straight. Return your leg against resistance to the starting position, and repeat. Switch legs. This exercise strengthens the hamstrings, gluteals, and erector spinae.

These exercises surely will improve your leg power and maybe will make you a better sprinter. But would they make you a better distance runner?

The same question troubled me. Concerned by my poor strength performance some years ago during a fitness test with *Aerobics* author Kenneth H. Cooper, MD, at the Cooper Clinic in Dallas, I returned home and consulted Charles Wolf, director of a physical therapy department in northwestern Indiana. Dr. Cooper's test showed I had little power for the leg and knee extensions, even for my age group. But he was measuring pure power, the kind that makes you a better sprinter or weight lifter. Wolf duplicated the tests, but added one more—a leg endurance test that involved 30 repetitions rather than just four, as used in Dr. Cooper's test. On the 30th rep, I was kicking with almost the same power as on the first. I had endurance.

But what about strength? "As a distance runner, you don't need a lot of strength," admitted Wolf. "You just need a little strength at the right time." The "right time" is the moment that the leg pushes off the ground, propelling the runner forward. That particular action is a functional strength, and it is best trained by running. For distance runners, therefore, weight training may be best as a supplemental activity.

> *It is hard to ignore the positive benefits runners consistently report from strength training.*

RUNNERS WHO BENEFIT MOST

Do you think your running would benefit from weight training? Certain individuals probably benefit more from strength training than others.

Ectomorphs. These are individuals considered to be of the slender physical type—"having a thin body build," my dictionary politely says. Ectomorph is the opposite of endomorph, someone with more muscle and a heavier body build. You know who you are, you ectomorphs. I'm one of you. When younger, I was effective as a runner because at peak training I weighed between 136 and 138 pounds. The most muscular part of my body was my legs. The front ranks of any distance race consist primarily of ectomorphs. Many, if not most, of these front-runners probably need to do at least some weight lifting to maintain their strength and speed—as long as they can do it without significantly increasing their bulk or weight.

Women. One of the main differences between men and women is strength. It's a simple fact of genetics. Thus, women probably can benefit more from strength training than men—as long as the extra strength does not equal extra weight. It is also important for women to build strength to limit their risk of bone disorders such as osteoporosis.

Masters. "Strength fades as we age," insisted the late Michael L.

Pollock, PhD, who was director of the University of Florida's Center for Exercise Science. (Before his death, Dr. Pollock supervised one of the most comprehensive longitudinal studies on the effects of exercise on aging.) "As strength fades, so does speed." It's easily measurable in the laboratory. As we move through the ages, from 30 to 40 to 50 and onward, we lose strength faster than endurance. That's one reason why older runners have more success in ultramarathons (races beyond 26.2 miles) than in 1500-meter races against younger runners. "As you get older, you need to focus more and more on this (strength) aspect of your conditioning," said Dr. Pollock.

George Lesmes, PhD, director of the Human Performance Laboratory at Northeastern Illinois University, notes that he has been able to increase

Genetics determines how many muscles we have.

the endurance of men 55 and older by offering them strength training for their legs. "They can stay up on the treadmill longer," says Dr. Lesmes, "and it's simply a matter of strength equaling improved endurance."

Given these examples, the person most likely to improve running speed through strength training would be a skinny female masters runner. (As a skinny male masters runner, I fit two of the categories, which is one reason I now put more emphasis on strength training.)

Kathy Morse, 51, a barber shop owner from Lowville, New York, agrees with me. Morse feels that as she gets older, strength training becomes more and more necessary: "I've been running for over 20 years, and to maintain my fitness levels I really need the strength training. I've noticed that as I run I'm able to carry myself easier, building my core strength has made such a difference."

Do these assessments mean that if you are a muscular young male, you need not worry about strength training? Not necessarily. More than likely, the benefits for you will be less, but that's no reason to shun the weight room. As you age (and we all do), the muscle you built while younger will continue to benefit you. In fact, the best time to build muscle mass and overall body fitness, whether you're male or female, is when you're young. Then, hang on to it!

GIVE STRENGTH A CHANCE

The rules are set: Muscle fiber cannot be created. Genetics determines how many muscles we have. Muscle fibers, however, can be thickened, an increase in size that is called hypertrophy. Exercise physiologist Dean Brittenham explains that lifting heavy loads (more weight, fewer repetitions) tends to build maximum strength and muscle size. Lifting less weight but with more repetitions develops greater muscle endurance, along with muscle definition. But competitive runners are not interested in muscle size or muscle definition, that pumped-up look that is more often reserved for bodybuilders.

I offer a popular Tip of the Day on Facebook that sometimes covers strength training. I follow the Brittenham approach, suggesting that runners focus on light weights and high repetitions rather than on heavy weights and few repetitions. Inevitably, this causes those who feel the other way to complain about my advice. "Bad thread," one antagonist posted recently. Sometimes, I click on the antagonist's name, which links me to their Facebook page, which more often than not shows pictures of bodybuilders.

Strength training, it seems, is a subject similar to religion or politics: You need to be careful what you say and to whom you say it. Gabriel Mirkin, MD, once wrote in *The Runner* magazine, "There is no proof that (lifting) will in any way improve your times." This caused a reader from New Jersey to reply: "Dr. Mirkin may be correct for runners blessed with a fair amount of upper-body strength," he wrote. "But I had very little strength to begin with and have found (after 6 months of Nautilus training) that I can now run any race without the extreme fatigue I formerly felt in my shoulders and arms."

It's a good point, but it proves only that strength training benefited that particular runner. It may not benefit all of us. So how do you know if weight training is right for you? Let's consider the subject further.

FIGHTING UPPER-BODY FATIGUE

Masters runner Bob Schlau is one who believes that strength training can improve speed. He told me about his own experience for an article I was writing on strength training for *Runner's World* magazine. Schlau claimed that prior to 1980, his arms and shoulders always tired toward the end of a race (usually a marathon). His legs also started moving more slowly, so his pace fell off. "My upper body would just go dead," he told me. "I know it affected my times."

Hoping to improve his performances, Schlau began a strength-training program for his upper body. He developed a 3-day-a-week routine of weight work that included situps, stretching, and free weights. "All upper-body

CORRECTING IMBALANCES

To both correct and prevent muscle imbalances, Julie Isphording, a competitor for the United States in the 1984 Olympics in Los Angeles, recommends strength training twice a week for 20 minutes, both lower and upper body, after running rather than before. "Running must remain your priority," says Isphording. "The best time to strength train is after your run, usually on an easy day."

For your lower body, specifically the muscles around the knees, Isphording recommends leg extensions. Use either a machine or place a weight on your ankle. When ready, slowly straighten your leg. Lunges also are good for strengthening the trunk. "With your shoulders back, take a lunging step forward, dropping your back leg toward the floor, then lifting up. Use hand weights to increase the stress," Isphording instructs. (Be sure your front knee doesn't extend over your foot.) To strengthen your abductors and adductors, do side lifts (raising the weighted leg sideways). Hamstrings can be best exercised using machines.

Crunches remain a good stomach-strengthening exercise, and planks are also a popular method to develop core strength. For your arms and shoulders, use machines, free weights, or dumbbells, which can be swung to simulate the running motion. In all weight-lifting exercises, concentrate on form.

"Ask a strength trainer for help if you don't know how to do the exercise," cautions Isphording.

stuff," Schlau said. "Mostly curls and presses. I also take light weights and replicate the running motion with my arms."

Did it work? Soon after starting his strength routine, Schlau found he no longer had trouble with arm and shoulder fatigue, and it improved his 5K and 10K times as well. At age 42, he ran a 30:48 10K. It is the contention of Dr. Becque, of course, that strength training is particularly important for masters like Schlau. "One of the first things you lose as you age is power," says Schlau.

Yet one of the most successful masters runners claimed he never weight trains. Norm Green, a minister from Wayne, Pennsylvania, won the 10,000 meters at both the 1987 and 1989 World Masters Championships. His 10,000 time in the 1989 meet in Eugene, Oregon, at age 57, was a rather incredible 33:00. I say incredible because I got a good look at him as he lapped me. Green is a naturally powerful, well-muscled runner. Yet he claimed to rely only on the basics. He just ran hard in every workout and rarely let his pace lag slower than 6 minutes per mile.

Would Norm Green benefit from strength training? The evidence suggests that Green ran fast enough without pumping iron. Has Schlau benefited from strength training? It's possible that his fast 10K times came from other aspects of his training, but I'm not about to suggest that Schlau walk away from the weight room. And I'm not asking Green to join Schlau. They're individuals. Each benefits from different types of training. Strength training may have little to no impact on one runner's performance, but may lead to significant improvements for another.

SEEKING ALL-AROUND FITNESS

To develop an all-around fitness program, Dr. Pollock suggested a minimum of 2 days a week of resistance training. Each session should last approximately 20 minutes and include 8 to 12 repeats on each of the major muscles of the body: legs, hips, trunk, back, arms, and shoulders. This work is in addition to a general aerobic program (such as running) that also should include warmup, stretching, and cooldown. "It's important to exercise all major muscle areas of the body," said Dr. Pollock. "Aerobics is good for legs and heart and body composition, but it won't strengthen muscles or maintain their strength, so a well-rounded program is very necessary."

Keep in mind that Dr. Pollock was more interested in developing fitness, not speed. Someone hoping to use strength training to run fast might like to try something like my own routine. Despite relatively low marks in the strength test at the Cooper Clinic, I have always incorporated weight training into my program. And I find it helps.

In 1958, I competed in the National AAU 30K Championships in York, Pennsylvania, and placed third. The main sponsor was the York Barbell Company, whose president, Bob Hoffman, was an avid fitness promoter. My prize was a pair of barbells.

For several years, I used the barbells on my back porch. This was during a period when I was a contender in every race I ran. (I placed fifth in the 1960 Olympic Trials in the 3000-meter steeplechase.) Untutored, I utilized the three Olympic lifts used in weight-lifting competition: three attempts at each lift to see how much iron I could throw over my head. (Don't even ask!) I also worked out occasionally in the weight room at the University of Chicago. That was rather unusual for a distance runner in those days, but at that time, I considered pumping iron as an important part of serious training.

Eventually, I donated my York barbells to Mount Carmel High School in Chicago, where I coached for several years in the mid-1960s. I drifted away from weight lifting for a decade as I took a hiatus from elite competition, then bought a set of weights for my son. When he went to college, I appropriated them.

In the mid-1970s, I became more and more involved in masters competition. I met Bill Reynolds, an Olympic lifting candidate who wrote *The Complete Weight Training Book*. We were both speakers at a clinic in California sponsored by *Runner's World* magazine. Reynolds, wisely, was cautious about promising benefits for distance runners. Nevertheless, he taught me five basic lifts that improved my overall fitness and athletic performance.

■ **Clean and press.** This is one of the Olympic lifts. Stand with your feet spread about shoulder-width apart. Reach down, grasp the bar, and bring

(continued on page 238)

TIPS FOR THE WEIGHT ROOM

Here are some things to keep in mind as you head to the weight room.

Running remains your best strength exercise. Exercise is very specific. To best develop your running muscles, you need to run—and run fast. Hill running is most favored by many runners interested in building strength. Weight lifting and other forms of strength training are important mainly as supplemental activities.

Don't compete with other lifters. The worst thing is to walk into a weight room and try to lift the same loads as weight-trained athletes around you. You wouldn't expect a 230-pound hunk to beat you in a 5K, so don't expect to outperform him in his sport.

Balance the benefits of free weights versus machines. Free weights do a better job of exercising the total body because they stress multiple muscles in a single lift. Machines, on the other hand, isolate muscle groups. If you choose to use free weights, be careful. Since they're not connected to a frame and pulleys, they can be dangerous if you're not accustomed to using them. Some lifts—such as squats and half squats—require proper lifting form to avoid injury risk, so seek out qualified instruction. The late Michael L. Pollock, PhD, who was director of the University of Florida's Center for Exercise Science, recommended exercise machines for masters because of safety. "As we age, we have balance problems," Dr. Pollock advised. "You're less likely to get hurt using a machine."

Avoid heavy weights. If you're interested in improving performance, as opposed to physique, stay away from lifting heavy weights. They may be hard on the lower joints, or they may cause you to bulk up. Excessive upper-body weight is dead weight in a 5K. Watch your bathroom scale. If your weight-lifting routine causes you to gain bulk, try using less weight with more repetitions. I know from the times when I have posted this advice online that not everybody agrees with me. The flaming begins. Will heavy weights improve your strength and thus your speed? Possibly, but I worry about rookie runner/lifters injuring themselves. If you want to lift heavy, please find a strength coach to supervise your training.

Don't try to peak as a weight lifter. Some strength coaches advise you to fatigue each muscle to its maximum, increasing weights and varying reps as you improve in strength. This might be on-target for building muscles and bulk, but as a runner, that is not your goal. Over a period of time, develop a strength workout that you can do comfortably and consistently. Stay with it. Don't feel you need to do more.

Vary your lifting. The hard/easy principle works in lifting as well as in running. Lifters typically work one group of muscles one day, then rest those muscles the next day while they exercise a different group. If you're lifting on a daily basis, you may want to do the same.

Lift on your easy days. Coming in from a grinding interval workout and heading for the weight room is not a great idea. Save your lifting for those days when you run at an easier pace. Even after your easy run, rest a bit before hitting the weights. Exercise physiologist Dean Brittenham suggests doing your strength training at a different time of day from when you run. He feels that way, you'll get more out of each workout. True, but not all of us want to commit the time necessary for double workouts.

Lift most during the off-season. Not every runner has an off-season, but the best time of year for strength training is when you are not training hard or racing often. For those of us in the North, that's usually in the winter; for those in the hot and humid South, it may be summer.

Don't overlook the value of calisthenics. Situps, pushups, and pullups remain effective means of developing and maintaining strength. You don't need to buy a high-tech machine or join a glitzy health club. You can include calisthenics as part of your regular stretching routine.

Be your own person. Eventually, each runner should develop a strength routine specific to his own needs. "Whether or not strength training makes you a faster runner," says David L. Costill, PhD, "it makes you a fitter individual."

it overhead in one continuous movement. Return the bar to the floor and repeat.

- **Bent-over row.** With your knees slightly bent to prevent stress on your back, reach down and grasp the bar with your palms facing down. Lift the bar to your chest without rising from the bent position. Return the bar to the floor and repeat.

- **Upright row.** Again, with your palms down, bring the barbell to an upright position so that you are standing straight, with the bar resting against the fronts of your thighs. Letting your elbows go out to the sides, raise the bar to chest height, keeping it close to your body. Repeat.

- **Curl.** This is a basic lift for any weight-training routine. Assume the same position as for the upright row, with the barbell resting against the fronts of your thighs. This time, though, your palms should be facing up instead of down. With your elbows close to your body, lift the bar to chest height. Repeat.

- **Military press.** Perhaps the most basic lift. In the upright position, with your palms down, bring the bar to shoulder height. Raise the bar over-head, fully extending your arms, then bring the bar back to shoulder height, and repeat.

Following Reynolds's advice, I did these routines with low weights and high repetitions. I stretched between sets of 10 and lifted only every other day—usually during the off-season, when I had no important races. Although I have significantly modified my strength-training routine in recent years, I continue to use these lifts from time to time and refer to them, at least mentally, when making any changes in my strength training routine.

MACHINE DISCIPLINE

At one time, my wife, Rose, played tennis at a local health club, so we had a family membership. When the club added a Nautilus center, I moved some of my training there. While Rose was snapping backhands, I pumped iron.

This was during a period when Nautilus ruled the weight rooms, both in machines and in advice on how to use those machines. The Nautilus approach was to begin at an easy level (much as you might in Week 1 of a marathon training program) and gradually increase the number of repetitions and weight lifted to reach a hard level (much as you might in Week 15 of a marathon training program). I have no argument with this approach, except I currently am more interested in maintaining strength/fitness rather than improving it, which may be the wisest approach for aging masters.

One distinct advantage of the machines you find in a gym is that you can focus on a specific muscle group and avoid stressing others. This is important when recovering from injuries. Unless you have some specific muscle imbalance, or your weight training is supervised by a strength coach who knows about running, you might want to avoid maxing out with too many reps or too much weight. You definitely do not want to develop antagonistic muscles that can interfere with your running stride.

While it's important to have strong quadriceps to get you through the last few miles of a marathon, bulky quads can be a hindrance. If you don't believe me, check the quads on cyclists who compete in the Tour de France. Their quads often are so large, they almost overlap their kneecaps. These athletes are very good at what they do—riding a bike very fast for endless hours—but running can be very painful for them.

Cross-training that includes strength training and other aerobic activities also can be a mixed blessing. Despite their overall athletic ability, few triathletes have great success in running-only races. No Ironman winner has won a major marathon, despite the lure of six-figure prize money. "Studies show that specificity of training is key to performance," says Dr. Costill. "If you want success as a runner, you need to focus almost all of your training on running and the muscles that allow you to run fast. If you want success as a triathlete, you need to balance your training for all three sports. Switching back and forth from sport to sport does not always work." Dr. Costill speaks as someone who was a champion masters swimmer, who held nine masters age-group records. In road races, he had a marathon best of 3:07, fast but nowhere near his swim accomplishments.

For a period of several years, I suffered what I called a "midlife triathlon crisis." As a break from running competition, I concentrated some of my energy on triathlons and was good enough one year to qualify for the Ironman triathlon in Kona, Hawaii (although I did not compete in that prestigious event). While training for three sports, I discovered that the faster I was able to ride a bicycle, the slower I was able to run. For every minute I took off my bike-leg time, I gained a minute on my running-leg time.

For this reason, I advise runners to be cautious about overdoing cross-training. (Notice I used the word "overdoing.") Despite my own disclaimers, I have begun to do more lap swimming as an alternate fitness activity. As I age, I discover I find it increasingly difficult to run as many miles as I once did. I need more rest days. Yet I enjoy the work break that exercise gives me. I spend too much time in front of a computer in my home office. Some days, if I don't get out to run, I don't get out of the house. At our local fitness facility, my wife participates in a water aerobics class, and I first pump iron in the gym, then head to the pool to swim laps and run laps in chest-deep water. I swim both to strengthen my upper body and to burn calories, whether or not it makes me a better runner. I always thought lap swimming had to be the world's most boring activity, but, surprisingly, I now find that I enjoy it.

Most of my cross-training and strength training is intuitive; very little is scientific. I do it as much because I enjoy the discipline as from any knowledge that it will improve (or maintain) my speed. I feel that extra strength does equal extra speed, but I can't prove it and apparently neither can most of the scientists with whom I consulted. Nevertheless, we all agree that strength training is an important activity that we all should do.

CHAPTER TWENTY-ONE

THE POLISHING TOUCH

Be your own best coach

One of the secrets of becoming a faster runner is learning not merely how to train but also when to train—in other words, putting it all together. In 1988, Lynn Jennings proved herself as one of the world's best runners. Self-coached, she placed sixth at the Olympic Games in Korea—no small accomplishment. But as Jennings herself admitted, "I had stalled out." She wanted to run faster.

"My goal," said Jennings, "wasn't just to be the best American runner; I wanted to be the best in the world." To achieve that goal, she began training the following April under the direction of John Babington, an attorney who coached for the Liberty Athletic Club in Cambridge, Massachusetts.

The combination clicked. In January 1990, Jennings set a world indoor record for the 5000 meters at the Dartmouth Relays. In February, she broke the American record for the 3000, winning the national Track and Field Championships. In March, she ran 31:06 for an American road record at the Red Lobster 10K Classic. And most famously, later that month, in Aix-les-Bains, France, she became the first American woman in 15 years to win the World Cross Country Championships.

"All changes should be gradual, not abrupt."

As Jennings already had demonstrated, she knew how to train. She also knew her own physiological strengths and weaknesses, having been tested frequently by expert scientists as a member of Athletics West, the Nike-sponsored club in Oregon. What Babington offered to Jennings was

WHY HIRE A COACH?

Most runners are self-coached, but sometimes they can improve their ability to run fast by seeking the advice of a coach. You can also get coaching advice by joining a team or an online training program. Here are 10 services that a coach can provide for a runner seeking improvement.

Motivation. Getting started is important for beginners; keeping going is a necessity for even experienced runners. A good coach can provide the necessary jump-start in the first case and continuous pushing in the latter. Reporting on a regular basis to a coach or mentor—even only once a week or by e-mail or phone—can provide an important keystone to any training plan.

System. Good coaches have been compared to chefs. They know how to mix the different ingredients. In addition to a system, they also have a methodology. Often, the details in any system are secondary to its mere existence.

Planning. Proper planning can sharpen the focus of your goals. A coach can help pick goals that are realistic and design training plans to achieve those goals, both long- and short-term.

Advice. Once a runner has been working with a coach for a long time, the training plan becomes obvious. One key role for coaches advising elite athletes is picking races, particularly knowing when to say no in this era of run for the money. But average runners need similar help to avoid overracing.

Injury prevention. Big plus. A coach who carefully monitors an athlete's progress can recognize when the athlete begins to show signs of the fatigue from overtraining that often precede any injury. But something that all runners need: organization, an objective look at her abilities, and advice on setting goals and peaking for important contests.

"One thing we did at the outset," recalls Babington, "was that we looked at what was her stable and comfortable level of training. It was a ballpark

even more important, a coach can help prevent overtraining, which often leads to injury.

Plateau busting. Sooner or later, all runners reach the point at which they fail to improve. How to get off a plateau is a common problem. A good coach can suggest different types of training that may allow the plateaued runner to climb upward to a new level of performance.

Checklist. A good coach provides a system and a plan to the relationship. The coach knows the athlete: his or her background, his or her potential. This allows the coach to prescribe workouts, not only for the day, but for weeks and months down the road. This allows the runner to focus on the actual training with an open mind.

Feedback. Most runners maintain logs or diaries, on paper or online, but they don't always know how to interpret accumulated information. A coach, based upon his experience with many athletes, can evaluate training from an unbiased point of view. Feedback, going both ways, is essential in the coach/athlete relationship.

Cheerleader. Runners' muscles run on glycogen, but their minds often run on praise. They need encouragement. A coach can offer a shoulder to cry on after a bad race or a pat on the back after a good race.

Fun. A coach can make training fun by offering a variety of workouts and running routes. The coaching environment offers an opportunity to interact with other runners working with the same coach. For those who run for enjoyment, this may be the best reason to hire a coach.

amount of mileage that involved a carefully chosen intensity. We asked ourselves, what components can we upgrade without exhausting her? What
additional training margin could she benefit from?

"There's a general principle that says if you want to get better, don't bite
off more than you can chew. All changes should be gradual, not abrupt. Our
starting point was based on Lynn's lifestyle and time constraints. We asked
ourselves, what one or two things can we change, or upgrade, to make her a
better runner?"

Let me interject a slight revision to that comment: What one or two *small*
things could Jennings and Babington change, or upgrade, to make her a better runner? If there is anything I have learned from all the athletes I have
coached over many decades, it is that you do not make sudden moves—unless
you are trying to escape a barking dog.

Jennings and Babington observed that her weekly mileage had been relatively low for a world-class runner, between 50 and 60 miles. They decided
to push into the 70s. Jennings benefited from this small shift in her training.
"That was one of the main differences between Lynn in 1988 and Lynn in
1990," Babington says.

Training adjustments often are achieved most easily with a coach riding
shotgun. The instinct of most runners when they want to improve is to do
more, but in some instances, they may be better off doing less. Not every runner is like Jennings, who found she needed to do more to develop an edge. As
head of the New York Road Runners Club's coaching program, Bob Glover
supervised 20 coaches, who in turn supervised hundreds of runners. "At the
beginner level," says Glover, "people benefit from being enrolled in a fitness
program, because they tend to do too much too soon. For individuals making
the transition into racing, a coach can encourage them. The faster a runner
gets, the less there is to push. At the elite level, runners have so much drive
they don't need a coach pushing them; they need a coach holding them back."

Coach Jim Huff of Detroit's Motor City Striders stresses the importance
of planning. "You need to look at your training program, determine specific
goals, and develop a program that will help you accomplish those goals, as
long as they are realistic. Unfortunately, a lot of runners don't have the basic
know-how to progress toward a goal."

THE COACH APPROACH

One way you can better plan your training is to obtain a coach—a Babington, Glover, or Huff—who can apply the generally accepted principles of training outlined in this book to your goals. Unfortunately, most runners don't have a coach and never will. I have mostly been self-coached during my career as both a semi-elite runner and a master. This was not entirely from self-choice. There simply was no knowledgeable coach nearby who I felt could assist me with my training. Moreover, this was at a time before the Internet as we know it today and the easy access it provides to online coaches.

Being self-coached, I've found that you don't always need a coach, but you do need to know coaching principles. Just as there are sound physiological principles involving aerobic and anaerobic training that can help you maximize performance, there also are sound coaching and planning principles that can help you succeed. In fact, the latter may be more important than the former.

Putting together your own coaching program just takes a little planning and the knowledge that you have gained from this book. Here are some suggestions that a good coach might offer you.

Plan Ahead

Exercise physiologist Edmund R. Burke, PhD, once said, "Good order is the foundation of all good things."

When Coach Babington sought improvement for Jennings, their first action was to sit down and plan her long-range training. I do the same for myself. Flying home from the World Masters Championships in Germany one year, I planned my training for the 18 months leading up to the next world meet. That was the first step to ultimately winning the gold medal at the championship in 1981.

Each year, I would review the previous year's results and plan ahead, determining what races to peak for—even determining whether I wanted to peak. Some years, I focused attention on short track races; other years, I shifted to the roads. I sometimes planned to take a year off, where I ran mainly for fun. But it's a conscious decision. You can't get where you're going without a road map.

Look Behind

You also can't get where you're going unless you know where you've been. Record your training on a daily basis. In my office in Indiana, I have a set of loose-leaf notebooks dating back to 1963, when I was fortunate to have the attention of two-time Olympian Fred Wilt as my coach. He asked me to record daily workouts on $5\frac{1}{2}$ by $8\frac{1}{2}$-inch diary sheets, which he provided. Later, I developed my own training diary sheet, which I had printed in large numbers for minimal cost. Much later, I used an interactive program to log workouts into my computer.

I would record items such as the date, time, location, surface and conditions, and distance, along with my weight. I also recorded what I did to warm up and cool down, and any comments concerning the actual run. There was space in my old diary sheets to record an optional second workout and boxes for race split times. (It's also a good idea to include space to jot down notes on your diet.) I also developed different diary formats for my cross-country ski workouts and for my high school team. Eventually revolutions in computer technology allowed me to save everything online.

There are several reasons for keeping a diary, whether or not it is digital or handwritten on paper. One, it provides motivation, the same way reporting your workouts to a coach would be motivational. Two, it allows you to learn from your successes and failures. If you ran well, what type of training was responsible for your success? If you ran poorly or were injured, what training error was responsible? I quickly learned that a weight between 136 to 138 put me in position to record great achievements. But if that weight slipped to 135 and below, something bad was about to happen.

Running logs are important equipment, almost as important as running shoes.

Define Your Goal

What do you want to accomplish with your running? Is it continued fitness and the enjoyment of staying in shape? If so, your training plan will differ from one designed to maximize your performance and to run fast times.

Most runners choose goals that are event-oriented. They desire to run well in a specific event—a local race, a national championship, a major marathon or half marathon. Event-oriented goals are helpful because they allow you to tie your training to specific dates.

But one coach I discussed this with warned against choosing too many goals. I was told that runners who simultaneously set ambitious goals at very different distances, say a sub-25 minute 5K *and* a sub-4 hour marathon, will probably fail to achieve either goal. Concentrate on one or the other to allow more precise planning. Pick one goal this season, then go after the other the next.

Be Realistic

If your fastest 10K time after several years of serious training is 45 minutes, you hardly should expect to break 30 minutes and qualify for the Olympic team within a year. Set your goals and plan your training conservatively. If you exceed your hopes, you can always aim slightly higher next time.

Bruce Tulloh, formerly one of Great Britain's fastest 5000-meter runners, writes in *Running*, "When building your own schedule, the first thing to decide is the volume of training which you can handle, both in total and in the number of good sessions a week. The training load you undertake must always be related to what you have been doing, not what you think you ought to do."

Don't Get Trapped

Historian Max Lerner once warned that we should learn from history but not be trapped by it. He was thinking of global issues such as war, but the advice is apropos for running, too. One of the dangers of having records for several decades of training on your shelves is believing that what worked once may work again. Some of my best training years were 1956, 1964, 1972, 1980, and 1991. I made breakthroughs or won championships in each of those years because of major shifts in my approach to training—sometimes more miles, sometimes more quality—but it is impossible for me to duplicate those workouts or workout patterns today. I approached my training differ-ently in each of those bonanza years, and I will continue to do so in the future.

Our bodies change. Our situations change. Our motivations change. We age. Everything is different. A particular danger is for someone who starts running again after a slack period of a dozen or more years to think he or she can train like he or she did in high school. There are a lot of other things you did in high school that you wouldn't—or shouldn't—do again. Be wise.

Make Smart Changes

Coach Babington suggested only one small adaptation to Jennings: Increase mileage. She added only 10 to 20 miles to her weekly total. Both coach and athlete realized that if she made too radical a shift in her training routine, they risked undoing all of her previous gains.

At one point in my career, I tried to increase the number of quarters in my interval workouts (going from 10 to 20) and to decrease the times (going from 70 seconds to 60). Before I could reach my goal of 20 repeats of 60-second 400s, I crashed. Years later, I reflected on this training mistake with Frank McBride, who was coaching me at the time. "We violated at least two of Gerschler's five training principles," he admitted. (See Chapter 13 for more about German coach Waldermar Gerschler and his theories on inter-val training.)

That's the kind of mistake you make only once if you're an intelligent runner. If you're superintelligent, or at least were smart enough to purchase a copy of this book, you'll avoid making it even once. In plotting your train-ing progression, concentrate on improving one area at a time—and go about it gingerly.

Get Out Of the Rut

Runners often get stuck on plateaus and fail to improve because they fail to change their training. Distance running will help you run faster; so will speedwork. But if you're stuck on one type of training to the complete exclu-sion of all others, you probably will fail to maximize your performance. One way to improve is to do something different, almost regardless of what that something is.

Be innovative. Change training sites. Join a different health club. Find a coach. Shift sports. If you're a track runner, you might benefit from doing some road running. Road racers probably should move to the track—or try cross-country. If your focus is marathons, try some 5Ks; if your focus is 5Ks, try a marathon.

At various times in my career, I've shifted more of my competitive focus to cross-country skiing or triathlons just to break the routine. There are many types of distance

In plotting your training progression, concentrate on improving one area at a time—and go about it gingerly.

running, including orienteering (running with compass and map) and biathlons (shooting and skiing). In recent years, trail races have become quite popular, with many of the participants focused on competing in picturesque—but challenging—surroundings, instead of some time on a stopwatch. Want to have people throw colored paint at you while you run past them; or if you like to wallow in the mud, there are now fun runs and obstacle races you can enter. You can have all sorts of running experiences. If you move from one discipline to another, it will provide new goals, if nothing else.

Program Some Rest

The hard/easy training pioneered by the late Bill Bowerman of the University of Oregon works well. By taking off an easy day or two, runners can come back on their hard days and run that much harder. As I age, I find I need to pay much more attention to this approach. David L. Costill, PhD, claims that muscle changes occur on the rest day following a hard training session, rather than on the hard day. If you work hard day after day, you eventually tear down muscle.

During the summer of 1984, I had a conversation with British ace Sebastian Coe about a month before he won the 1500 meters and placed second in the 800 meters at the Olympic Games in Los Angeles. Coe was then 27; he had just torn through an incredible workout of 20 × 200 meters, averaging

27 seconds, resting only 25 to 45 seconds between each. He ran his final one in 22.5, a time good enough to win at least most high school 200 races. It was a mind-boggling workout, but afterward, Coe commented that several years earlier, when he was 20 or 21, he could do quality sessions such as that 4 or 5 days in a row. "Now that I'm older, I need more rest," he said, straight-faced.

"Most athletes will find that two hard sessions and one race per week is as much as they can take, with the other days being easy running for recuperation," says Tulloh.

Respect Your Environment

If you wake up in the morning and find the street in front of your house covered with a sheet of ice from a freezing rain, that's probably not the day to head to the track for a workout of repeat quarters—unless that track is indoors. Obviously, everybody needs to take note of the weather for specific workouts. But the best way to prepare for weather is to plan well in advance.

Living in the Midwest, having gone to college in Minnesota, I knew that winter offered a good period for long aerobic runs. I was forced to run slowly while wearing several layers of clothes and picking my way across icy patches or puddles in the road. Spring, I also knew, was a good time for fast anaerobic runs, since the footing is good and the weather's still cool. Summer was a time for repetition running, since I could pause between fast bursts to cool down or even take a drink. Autumn was similar to spring when it came time to run fast, plus it was a great time to run trails with leaves changing on the trees. But this scenario wouldn't necessarily hold true for a runner in Arizona or Alaska. When in Florida, I need to rethink my training to take advantage of the warmer winter weather plus the availability of a smooth and flat beach for training sessions. In planning your training, you have to be aware of the environment in which you run.

Progress Carefully Toward Your Goal

To improve with each performance, you need to carefully and progressively adapt your training. This is the principle of overload, whose historic innovator, the ancient Greek wrestler Milo, used to get stronger each day by lifting onto his shoulders a calf that eventually became a bull. When we increase our mileage on a daily or weekly basis, we essentially are doing the same thing.

But a lot of, well, bull is offered to runners about how they should progress. Some theories say to increase mileage by 10 percent a week or to run interval quarters a second faster each week. I don't believe in formulas. As you progress, make certain that you do so conservatively. But do progress.

Put It in Writing

One way to motivate yourself is visually, with either a chart or a poster on your wall. If your goal is a specific race time, maybe you should pass those numbers every day when you go out to train.

I'm a big believer in visual aids. One year, I designed my schedule for the season by drawing a calendar with 8 months of dates. On it, I outlined in red my scheduled mileage for

As you progress, make certain that you do so conservatively. But do progress.

each week and the race dates where I wanted to hit my peak. Using pins, I attached the calendar to a cork wall in my basement, where I do my stretching and weight training. I passed that chart every day when I left to run and when I returned. I scribbled mileage and times on it, too, in addition to recording them in my training log. That let me know whether I was still on schedule with my planned training.

Having a visual reminder of your goals and the training needed to attain them can help motivate you. Many runners use the training schedules for marathons and other distances noted on my Web site. A number of these runners have told me how they download the schedules and post them where they can see them every day. If you use a digital training log, consider setting reminders for important dates and training milestones.

Review Regularly

By reviewing my plans from time to time, I discover whether my original planning was overly optimistic. If it's April and my longest run over the past 3 months was 12 miles, but I plotted 18 miles for that date, I realize I may need to take a more realistic look at my plans and my goals. It may be time to return to the first tip on this list: Plan ahead.

CHAPTER TWENTY-TWO

READY TO RACE
Test your ability to run fast

Many runners fail to recognize the value of a thorough warmup. While competing one year in the Fall Frolic, a 4-mile race in Hammond, Indiana, I noticed that only a few of the participants took the time to warm up; probably a minority of that minority warmed up well. Sure, a number of runners popped out of the gym 15 or 20 minutes before the start on what admittedly was a cold and windy day to briefly jog up and down the street, but I suspect that was the extent of the warmup for most.

Warming up is a rarely discussed technique when it comes to running fast. And it's made complicated by the fact that so many runners fanning the flames of the fitness boom today never participated in track in high school, where they might have been coached in the values of the warmup. Everybody seems to know how to stretch (an art learned by watching others), but that's only part of a good warmup. (See also "A Great Warm-Up" on page 183 and dynamic flexibility techniques starting on page 189).

How important is a good warm-up? It probably won't lower your race time by more than a few seconds, let's say 5 to 10 seconds. That seems inconsequential over the length of a 10K race that might take you 45 minutes—unless you are shoulder-to-shoulder with some running buddy you've wanted to beat for the past 4 years. But let's face facts: You would not be reading this book if you did not want to shave every possible second off your times. At the elite level, hundredths of a second can make a difference of thousands of dollars, maybe even millions of dollars if you add endorsements to prize money.

There are numerous reasons to warm up correctly. First, a correct warm-up routine is valuable for preventing injuries. Cold muscles are more likely to pull than warm muscles. Then there's the matter of comfort. You can run more relaxed when your body is warm than when it's cold. The first mile or so of running never feels comfortable, not even for the most experienced runners, but you can raise your comfort level with a good warm-up. The athletic body simply functions better with its temperature raised a bit higher than normal. Minor irritations such as side stitches are less likely to occur if you warm up before going to the starting line. And since psychological considerations often overshadow physical talents when it comes to success, a good warm-up can focus your mind as much as your body. By warming up thoroughly, you signal your body that this is a day for running fast.

Of course, warming up can seem like an inconvenience. You need to get to the start earlier than you might otherwise. At many races, getting an adequate warm-up is difficult, if not impossible. At major races with tens of thousands of entrants, you may be forced to go to the line way too early to secure a spot in the starting corral. This can be quite a handicap, particularly for a short race. In a marathon, you often can start slow, planning to warm up gradually over the first few miles. But you can't afford to start too slowly in shorter races. It's a simple fact of racing life: The shorter the race, the faster the pace, and the warmer your muscles need to be at the start to reach full speed rapidly.

Certainly, the warm-up is most important in race situations because you go from standing still to full speed within seconds after hearing the starter's gun. But a full warm-up with stretching should not be overlooked during training either, particularly on those hard days when you run fast repetitions on the track.

The warm-up is particularly important for running in cold weather, when the temperature falls below 50°F and you don extra clothes to retain body heat. On the other hand, don't assume that you can skip the warm-up during warm weather because you are hot and sweaty. Pay special attention to the warm-up on those days when you feel you need it the least. Your muscles still need the extra performance boost that warm-ups deliver.

All told, the warm-up is a subject to which every runner should give full consideration. So as we reach the end of this book, let's do just that, beginning with warming up before workouts and later considering prerace warm-ups.

WARM-UP BEFORE WORKOUTS

Few runners have time to spend an hour warming up before their daily workouts. Even for races, warming up often seems more trouble than it is worth. Nevertheless, the faster you plan to run, the more you need to warm up. Here's how to do it right.

Make It a Habit

When I coached high school runners, I tried to instill good warm-up habits, which is not easy to do. Like herding cats? Not quite, but close. One problem is that every runner needs to find a warm-up routine to suit his or her rhythm. Unfortunately, team unity prohibits two dozen runners warming up two dozen different ways, particularly in cross-country, where the team usually tours the course as part of their warm-up. In track, runners more often can warm up on their own, since they compete in different events.

At the beginning of the season, I set aside one workout where we practiced warming up and nothing else. Similarly, for workouts the day before an important race, we would warm up only. Adult runners should give warm-ups careful attention, too. In the final 3-day countdown before a major race, such as a marathon, I usually prescribe two rest days and one easy-run day, that day actually being the day *before* the race. (For instance, an easy-run Saturday before a Sunday race.) For that Saturday workout, what better to do than a half hour or so devoted entirely to warm-up? Such an approach is particularly important if you just climbed off an airplane the day before.

Can a proper warm-up help you avoid injury? Can it make you a faster runner? That's difficult to prove scientifically, but I do believe the answer to both questions is, yes. A proper warm-up and cooldown should limit the damage you can do to your body, particularly when used before and after the intense workouts that are the heart of any program designed to help you run fast.

There are three components to my workout warm-up, which I also stressed to my high school runners. These steps are simple, and they can help prepare your muscles for a productive workout. One, I jog for 10 to 20 minutes. Two, I go through my stretching routine, as I describe in the next section. And three, my final step, I do a set of three or four easy sprints of 50 to 150 meters. All this serves to awaken my muscles.

Stretch for Success

Stretching is a subject that has launched a thousand magazine illustrations in *Runner's World* alone, but most runners probably can figure out how to stretch on their own or by watching other runners. If you want to learn from a book, Bob Anderson's classic *Stretching* remains in print after decades on the market.

Add to that all of the information available on the Internet. Googling the words "stretching exercises," I encountered 118 million entries in 0.42 seconds. I also learned from the American Running Association that I should, 1. never stretch a cold muscle; 2. use static stretching; 3. don't bounce or lunge; 4. breathe relaxed and naturally; 5. never stretch to the point of pain; 6. ease into and out of the stretch slowly and rhythmically; and 7. concentrate on how you feel in the stretch. Sounds pretty basic. You don't need to know too much more in order to teach yourself how to stretch. Of course, hiring a personal trainer or joining a class might teach you how to do it right.

I developed my own standard stretching routine over a period of time, without any particular scientific basis other than it felt good. I suggest you approach stretching from the same point of view. The purpose of stretching preworkout, prerace, or pre-anything is to make you feel good as well as to get loose. Don't do some exercise just because you saw it on the Internet or because every other runner you know stretches that way. If it doesn't work for you, don't do it.

Having said that, let me tell you that most of my stretches flow from one to another. That wastes less time, which is important if you have a limited period for a stretching routine. Here's the Higdon list of stretches.

1. **Overhead reach.** Stand with your feet slightly spread and reach over-head. Focus on your posture and reach for the sky. Personally, I enjoy another version of this stretch. When I run to the nearby golf course, there's a favorite evergreen tree with a branch just within reach. I hang from it and enjoy the aromatic smell of the tree. But you can stand any-where that you find enough ground space and do this stretch. It's my opener.

2. **Hang 10.** Stand with your feet slightly spread, bend forward from the waist, and let your fingers dangle toward the ground. The farther your legs are spread, the easier it is to touch the ground. But there is no shame in not touching. If some other runner tells me my knees are slightly bent, I ask them how fast they ran their last 10K. Unless it was 5 minutes faster than my time, I don't listen to their advice. Again, do what works best for you.

3. **Twist and turn.** Still standing, put your hands on your hips, bend at the waist, and rotate slowly—forward, sideways, and back. Do a few rotations in the clockwise direction, then in the counterclockwise direction. Wait a minute, isn't stretching supposed to be static? I'll check my rule book and text you the answer.

4. **Heel hold.** Support yourself with one hand on a wall or tree and grasp your ankle with the other hand, pulling it toward your buttocks. There are two ways to do heel holds. One way is to grasp your left ankle with your right hand, then your right ankle with your left hand. The other way is to grasp your left ankle with your left hand, then your right ankle with your right hand. Various experts have written why one heel hold is superior to the other. I sometimes do one, sometimes the other, some-times both, sometimes neither. Do whatever feels best for you.

5. **Wall lean.** Every runner knows this one. It's a safe, effective way to stretch your calf muscles. Find a wall or a stationary object such as a tree,

and stand about 2 feet away from it. Keep your heels planted firmly on the ground and place your hands on the wall, shoulder-width apart. Keeping your back straight, bend your elbows and gently lean forward. It feels good, plus it's an excellent stretch before fast races, where the calf muscles come into play.

There are a couple of variations on the wall lean. One is to lean with both feet together; another is to lean with one foot forward (knee bent) and one foot back, then switch. Take your pick.

A massage therapist I visited in Duluth, Minnesota, following Grandma's Marathon taught me an interesting variation of the split-leg wall lean. After stretching in one position, you move the front foot left and right, which stretches slightly different muscle combinations.

To stretch your calf muscles without a wall, stand tiptoe on stairs, allowing your heels to hang over the edge. Do the same going up escalators, too. Never miss an opportunity for a good stretch. Here are some more.

6. **Hurdle.** Sit on the floor with your legs in front of you. Bend your left leg to the side and keep your right leg straight in front of you. Support yourself with your left hand and reach for your toes with your right. Reach only as far as comfortably possible, without any pain. Don't force this stretch. After you've stretched your right leg, switch your position to stretch your left leg. To do this stretch effectively, try to picture what a track athlete looks like going over the 400-meter hurdles. It is okay to bend your front leg slightly; no need to press it against the ground. Since my signature event in track was the 3000-meter steeplechase, this was the most important stretch in my repertoire.

7. **Butterfly.** While you're sitting on the floor, put your legs straight out in front of you. Bend your knees so that they are pointing out to the sides and your feet are touching sole to sole. In this position, wrap your hands around your feet and press outward with your arms against the inside of your thighs, extending the stretch.

8. **Knee pull.** Lie flat on your back, and with your knee bent, bring one leg toward your chest, assisting it by pulling with both hands just below the

knee. Do the same with your other leg. I've been doing this stretch for years for no other reason than it feels good, but I saw the stretch pictured in a *Runner's World* article titled "An Ounce of Prevention." I must be on the right track.

9. **Horizontal reach.** This stretch is just like the overhead reach, the first stretch in this list, except you lie on your back. Point your toes and reach above your head with your fingertips. Hold the stretch for as long as it feels comfortable, then roll over and do the horizontal reach again, this time facedown. This is a comfortable stretch that I feel I could hold forever, but I seldom maintain a stretch as long as the de rigueur 30 seconds recommended by other experts.

10. **Belt-down pushup.** I use this pushup variation not to strengthen my arms but to loosen my back. The position is the same as for regular pushups, except that your lower body (your belt) remains "nailed" to the ground and you push up only the upper body. I usually do about five of these.

11. **Starter's crouch.** Few distance runners will find themselves in this position in a race situation, but I find it an effective stretching exercise. Pretending you're Usain Bolt at the start of the 100 meters, rise into a set position, but with the back leg fully extended. This gives you another variation on the wall lean. (But don't attempt to press your heel flat on the ground.) Switch legs, hold the stretch, then switch legs back and forth rapidly—a dynamic stretch. Remember, I don't limit myself to static stretches.

This ends the floor portion of my stretching routine. I rise and repeat one or two of the standing stretches with which I began my routine, most often the overhead reach or the twist and turn. If time is short, I may skip some stretches.

Can I complete almost a dozen stretches, some of them involving several variations, in 5 to 10 minutes? Sure. Each stretch flows from one to the other, and I hold each only as long as I feel comfortable. This way, I don't waste time. I'm not out to set an endurance record for stretching; I'm out to stretch to get ready for a comfortable, productive run. I follow my workout with an easy jog to cool down. It helps prevent injuries and keeps me in top form for racing.

A Final Warmup

Let me tell you about my personal warmup routine before a specific race, whether track race or road race. I like to arrive 60 to 90 minutes before race time. Sometimes, I'll cut it closer for a race I'm treating mostly as a hard workout (a summer fun run, for example), but an hour is almost minimal for any race in which I hope to perform well.

One plus in arriving early: You won't have to waste as much time standing in lines. If it is a major race with an expo the day before, you can arrive with your number already pinned to your singlet. If you need to pick up that number on race day, or even enter last minute, allow more time.

On some occasions, I'll do a prewarm-up at home before climbing into the car to go to the race. This prewarm-up may be less than a mile, just enough to loosen my bowels so I can visit the toilet before leaving for the race. And in the last few minutes of my drive, I'm still scouting for hidden toilets without people standing in line. You can waste a good warmup by being forced to stand in line for 10 to 15 minutes because the race organizers failed to provide adequate restroom facilities. A friend of mine used to joke about coming out of the porta-potty then immediately getting back into the same line for a second visit.

One advantage that road races have over track meets is that you can predict with some certainty the time the race will begin. If the entry blank announces an 8:00 a.m. start, a well-organized race will begin precisely at that time. At track meets, the mere number of scheduled races often causes delays, or races start earlier than stated, which is sometimes worse. Track runners often need to be more adaptable about their warm-ups than road runners.

60 MINUTES AND COUNTING

Sixty minutes before race time, I usually start my countdown. I try to use the same routine before each race, certainly before the important ones, because it is a routine that works for me. Here's how it goes. You are welcome to adopt this routine as your own, but you eventually may want to modify it, depending on your own preferences.

Jog (10 to 20 minutes). How far I go in my prerace jog depends on how loose I feel arriving at the start. A drive of more than an hour to the race, or hard training the week before from which I haven't fully recovered, may require me to spend more time and warm up more slowly. Generally, I like to go a couple of miles before most races. If I'm familiar with the area, I may jog to a location where I do the remainder of my warmup alone. It depends partly on how much the race means to me. Before important races, I may not want to waste my concentration chatting with other runners.

Relax (5 to 10 minutes). If I have not yet picked up my number, now is the time I do it. This may be time for another visit to the toilet, although everybody else usually has the same idea at this time.

Stretch (5 to 10 minutes). I try to find some quiet area (not always easy at large races) where I have enough room to stretch without being disturbed by too many people. If it's warm, I prefer to stretch outdoors on the grass, under the shade of a tree. As with my workout warmup, I begin with standing stretches, move to floor stretches, and finish by repeating some of the standing stretches. With 30 minutes left, I usually have finished stretching. At this point, I move into the next phase of my warm-up.

Flexible play (5 to 10 minutes). This is a dynamic extension of my stretching routine that includes bounding and strides, with jogging and walking in between. I don't utilize my full set of bounding exercises, but do two or three at the most. High knees and high heels are handy because they are simple and less stressful. (See "High Knees" on page 191 and "High Heels" on page 192.) But try them out in your workouts first. Don't include bounding in your race warmup unless you bound regularly as part of your training.

More essential are the strides. Run three or four easy sprints of 50 to 150 meters at a pace not much faster than your race pace to remind your legs about the task at hand. I like to accelerate very gradually, hit a good pace in the middle, then gradually decelerate. I walk and jog between strides. Before a road race, I pick out a straight section of street for this routine. If possible, I choose a stretch that slants slightly downhill, doing my fast strides that way because it makes me feel faster. For the same reason, I always run my strides downwind.

In teaching warmup routines to his team at Southwestern Michigan College in Dowagiac, coach Ron Gunn had his athletes do a 200-meter run at race pace exactly 20 minutes before race time. I've followed this approach on occasion and feel it works particularly well on those days when nothing you do seems to loosen you up. Just pushing that extra distance at a fast pace seems to help. Yes, you'll use energy that you may otherwise have conserved for the race, but in 5K and 10K races, energy conservation is not usually the problem. You should have ample energy for the job at hand; if a long stride during the prerace warm-up aids your ability to get loose, go for it.

Another variation on this routine is to run three strides of increasing length: 20, 30, and 40 seconds, or 100, 150, and 200 meters.

Final preparations (10 to 15 minutes). I've finished my warm-up. What remains is to get ready to race. Usually, I wait until now to don my racing singlet, preferring to go to the line with a dry shirt rather than one that's wet with sweat. On a cool day, I want to avoid getting even slightly chilled and losing the benefits of the warm-up. Also, I warm up in training shoes, then change to my lighter racing flats, or spikes. And I carefully knot my shoelaces to prevent them from coming untied midway through a race.

In the last few minutes, I jog easily and maybe take one or two more very short strides or stretch some more. Waiting for the gun,

I let my arms hang and shake my wrists in a last-minute battle with my nerves.

At high school races in Indiana, the starter often tells the runners to "shag out," meaning they are to sprint off the line for 50 to 75 meters, then gather in a circle to give a team cheer before jogging back to the start. But the dynamics of most road races rarely permit shag-outs by large numbers of runners. So I suggest you simply wait patiently, with the knowledge that, having followed the warm-up routine in this chapter, you are as hot to trot as anyone else in the field. The gun sounds. And you're off.

IS THAT ALL THERE IS?

Almost as fast as it starts, the race is over. You've crossed the finish line, and hopefully, you've sliced a few seconds off your old PR. You're ready to go home now, right? *Wrong!* There's one more thing left to do—your cooldown.

A cooldown obviously won't aid you in running the race just completed, but it will help you recuperate more rapidly. It helps you return to regular training more quickly, resulting in a stronger performance the next time you race. Thus within 5 minutes after crossing the finish line, I begin my cooldown at the same pace as my warm-up jog, but at half the distance. On cool days, I wear sweats. On warm days, I won't wait to change. As long as it doesn't interfere with the other runners, I like to turn around and jog back over the course, since it gives me an opportunity to see my friends finish. Sometimes I turn around and meet them at the line so we can cool down together. This is the beginning of the social hour.

Various people believe that we cool down to help process the removal of lactic acid and other waste products that may have pooled in our muscles during the final anaerobic sprint. This, they say, will prevent muscle soreness. That's only partially true. Lactic acid largely disappears within a half-hour, whether or not you do a cooldown. The soreness and stiffness experienced after a race is more from minute muscle fiber tears—micro tears, the experts call them—than from lactic acid.

(continued on page 266)

DETRAINING AND RETRAINING

Not everybody runs at the same level year after year after year. We move from peaks to valleys, gearing up for a road race and gearing down when other interests take precedence. Sometimes, we become injured. Sometimes, we become bored. Sometimes, we quit running (or run less) rather than fight the winds of winter or the dog days of summer. When we return back to the 5K or marathon, sometimes we encounter troubles.

Scientists now can describe the effects of detraining, or how quickly we go out of shape. At the University of Texas at Austin, Edward Coyle, PhD, convinced a group of highly trained runners (who ran 80 miles a week) and cyclists (who rode 250 miles a week) to quit training. Their measured oxygen uptake scores declined rapidly at first, then less so. Ironically, the best trained lost the most. Those less trained had less to lose. Dr. Coyle determined that athletes lost half of their aerobic fitness within 12 to 21 days, then half of their remaining fitness level within the next 12- to 21-day period, and so on. After 3 months, all were detrained.

Scientists find it more difficult to measure retraining, or how long it takes to get back in shape. "There's very little data," conceded the late Michael L. Pollock, PhD, who was director of the University of Florida's Center for Exercise Science. Nevertheless, scientists can make some educated guesses.

Dr. Coyle suggests that for every week lost, it takes 2 weeks to regain the original level of fitness.

In Dr. Coyle's detraining studies, he identified one reason for the immediate fitness decline—loss of blood volume. During the first 12 to 21 days away from training, you lose as much as a half-quart (500 milliliters) of blood. "Previously, researchers thought detraining was because of deterioration of the heart. Actually, the heart had less blood to pump to the muscles," states Dr. Coyle.

When you retrain, you regain that lost blood volume. Not only can you transport oxygen to the muscles more efficiently again, but you also have more fluid available for sweating, which helps cool your body. Dr. Coyle says runners can regain blood volume within a week, although reproduction of red blood cells takes longer.

But not all systems of the body detrain or retrain equally. Your skeletal system, for instance, may not accept the strain of training at your previous level, particularly as you age. Remember, a runner who loses 6 years of training must also cope with 6 years of normal aging.

Retraining need not be that difficult. And it is certainly easier than starting to run for the first time. If you are returning to running after being away for whatever reason, the following tips may make your journey back more pleasant.

Have a goal in mind. A goal may be as simple as going out to do your first run. Ask yourself why you want to run again. To get in shape? To improve your previous times? To compete in a particular race? Plan your training well ahead so as to achieve that goal.

Consider how long you've been gone. Depending upon your time away from fast training, you will have an easy or hard time coming back. Expect to spend at least 2 days getting back in shape for every day lost.

Forget the past. Workouts done years ago bear no relevance to what you can do today—and can be a cause of injury. Once you regain your base fitness, ask yourself whether you want to resume old training patterns, including speedwork.

Decide if you can do it better this time. In your previous life as a runner, did you make mistakes that can be avoided this time? Reevaluate your entire approach to training. Don't get trapped in old habits that maybe didn't produce the best results.

Consider your age. Runners in their twenties can head back to the track as though they never took any time off. It becomes progressively more difficult to regain lost speed once into your thirties, forties, fifties, and beyond. But it's not impossible.

Approach speedwork cautiously. Some speedwork seems necessary to regain peak performance. But until you rebuild your aerobic base, intense running may cause excessive fatigue and discourage you. Your tendons and ligaments may not support the new power developed by your lungs and muscles.

(continued)

DETRAINING AND RETRAINING–CONT.

Recognize that strength returns slowest. Just as strength is slowest to fade when you stop running, it takes longest to return. You will find it toughest to regain the top end of your conditioning, even when you're back in reasonably good shape.

Don't race too soon. Competition can be a good way to measure your comeback, but you risk injury by going too hard. It also takes time away from training. Go into early races with a relaxed mood, and don't worry about fast times.

Be cautious. If you've previously been injured, you should be particularly cautious. One important question to ask: "Have I determined the cause of the injury?" Rest is sometimes not enough. You may reinjure yourself if you train at your previous level.

Keep the faith. At times, it may seem the road back is too long to travel. But you can move back to road racing and perform at a high level. All it takes is discipline and patience.

A cooldown is a fun way to cap the experience. It gives you time to think about your race, and time to share it with others, if you like.

The better shape you are in, the more you will enjoy this social time. In fact, that's one benefit of running short races. I've never been able to do much immediately after a marathon, other than stare at the cup of yogurt in my hand and wonder how I'm going to summon enough energy to walk back to my hotel clad in a silly aluminum blanket. But 5 minutes after most shorter races, I'm ready to run again. Hopefully to run the next race faster than the one just finished.

Acknowledgments

A half century with Runner's World

The year was 1965, and I was at the peak of my powers. The previous year, I had finished as the first American in the prestigious Boston Marathon, just ahead of John J. Kelley, arguably America's finest long-distance runner for the previous decade. That summer of 1965, I out-kicked Kelley in the final mile of a major 25K race that started and finished on the grounds of the New York World's Fair. Also back in the field was a young Amby Burfoot, who, in 1968, would go on to win the Boston Marathon and serve later as executive editor for *Runner's World*.

Other than Boston, the media usually ignored road runners, but the win was important enough that the *New York Times* covered my victory the next morning, offering a photo taken postrace of our family: Rose and me and our three children, Kevin, David, and Laura. As Kevin stands dutifully aside, I hold his younger siblings in my arms, being properly smooched by Laura. Their mom's hair has been caught by the wind, creating a spiked 'do, still fashionable today. Rose looks absolutely gorgeous. Still does today. Many years later, David would hunt down a copy of the photo and offer it as a gift. The picture of our nuclear family hangs today in the hallway leading to the master bedroom of our condo in Ponte Vedra Beach, Florida.

The year 1965 was peak because, with the help of my coach, two-time Olympian Fred Wilt, I finally had figured out the training that took me—at least for a brief moment in time—to the top ranks of American long distance runners. Those who have followed my writings in magazines and books and on the Internet probably think that I sprung from the womb writing training programs, but it was far from that. It took me time to find out how to train. I had success as a track athlete in the 1950s, my best event the 3000-meter steeplechase in which I had placed fifth at the 1960 Olympic Trials, but the transition from track and field to road running did not go well for me. Arrogantly, I assumed that the same sort of training (mostly interval training) that worked in one branch of our sport would work in the other. It did not, and there was no *Runner's World* at the beginning of the 1960s to tell me otherwise. But eventually, thanks to Fred Wilt, I came up with the blend of speed, distance, and rest that is at the heart of all my training programs today. Unfortunately, I was in my mid-thirties when this happened, meaning that, no matter how hard I trained, I was going to get slower rather than faster as I moved through my forties and fifties and into my sixties and seventies and finally into my eighties, where I lodge now.

But looking back, 1965 was the top of the mountain. Soon after my New York victory, I received an invitation to the prestigious Kosice Marathon in Czechoslovakia. Kosice at that time was the unofficial world championships, bringing together the best runners from Western Europe and the best runners from Eastern Europe, plus at least in that year one runner from North America, me. The invitation, however, only covered my travel expenses from London to Kosice. Fortunately, being a full-time freelance writer, I knew how to scramble and convinced *Sports Illustrated* to let me write a feature article about the London to Brighton Race (an ultramarathon), featuring American Ted Corbitt. That would more than cover the first half of my expenses.

Alas, Kosice did not go well for me. I came down with a case of food poisoning two days before the race, causing severe dehydration. Up with the leaders for a while, I faded badly in the final miles, finishing 21st overall. Also disappointing, my article on London to Brighton got bounced out of the next issue of *Sports Illustrated*, and the issue after that and, lacking timeliness, never did run, although the magazine charitably paid full price for it.

A year later, I received a letter from a high school cross-country runner in Kansas City named Bob Anderson. At that time, there were two small-circulation magazines serving the running world: *Track & Field News* and *Long Distance Log*. Both focused mainly on results. Anderson came up with the unique idea of publishing a magazine that featured stories about the sport along with training information. He called his magazine *Distance Running News*. Its first issue, published in January 1966, sold out at 1,000 copies. This shocked many of us who were surprised that there even were that many distance runners in North America.

Anderson invited me to write for *Distance Running News*. He offered no money; he had very little to offer. Being a snooty professional journalist, I might have told him no. But I had that unpublished article about London to Brighton Race sitting in my files. I sent the article to Anderson, who used it on the front cover of the second issue of *Distance Running News,* which appeared later in July 1966.

And so began my half-century association with what would become *Runner's World* magazine, which is celebrating its 50th anniversary as I write these words.

Success came rapidly for Bob Anderson. Circulation climbed, forcing him to drop out of Kansas State University. He moved to the West Coast and hired Joe Henderson as editor. At the 1968 Olympic Games, I introduced Henderson to Dr. George Sheehan, whose monthly column of philosophy, not medicine, contributed to the success of the expanding magazine, which in 1970 was renamed *The Runner's World*.

Anderson's timing could not have been better. In 1972, Frank Shorter won the Olympic Marathon. In 1976, Jim Fixx wrote *The Complete Book of Running,* which sold a million hardback copies. Road races, which a decade earlier might have attracted a few dozen runners, now attracted a few thousand runners. One could say that Anderson's little magazine benefited from the running boom or you could say that he created the running boom. In truth, it was a little bit of both.

When New York publisher George Hirsch created a rival magazine, called *The Runner,* I began writing for him. Eventually Rodale, the health and fitness publishing giant located in Emmaus, Pennsylvania, purchased the two magazines and merged them into a single magazine. Under the direction of David Willey and his great team including John Atwood,

Runner's World gained a circulation of near 750,000. Because of the magazine's success, a lot of people read my books and take advantage of training advice that I wish I had while trying to make a stumbling transition from track and field to road racing all those years ago. Today, runners benefit from my advice not only in print but also online: Facebook, Twitter, my Web site, halhigdon.com. TrainingPeaks, headquartered in Boulder, Colorado, offers interactive versions of all my programs. Gear Fischer and Jeremy Duerksen head that operation. Bluefin, located in South Bend, Indiana, provides app versions you can download so that you can hear me talk to you as you run. Alex and Tanya Stankovic provide those products.

All of the people mentioned here contributed to my success as both a runner and as a journalist who writes about running. That includes those individuals at Rodale, such as Mark Weinstein, Franny Vignola, Sean Sabo, and Chris Gaugler, who served as key people in bringing *Run Fast* into its third edition. Credit also goes to my agent and close friend, Jan Seeley, who also serves as director of the Illinois Marathon.

Little did I realize 50 years ago in 1965 when, after winning a 25K at the New York City World's Fair and posing with my family for a photo that would appear in the next morning's edition of the *New York Times*, that a sport that attracted only a few hundred runners in even its most popular races would grow into a sport with millions of participants not only in the United States, but all over the world. *Runner's World* in this year of 2016 is celebrating its 50th anniversary, and I take great pride in saying I was with them right from the beginning. (Well, the second issue, if not the first.)

May all of us continue to run fast.

About the Author

Hal Higdon has contributed to *Runner's World* for longer than any other writer, an article by him having appeared in that publication's second issue in 1966. Author of more than three dozen books, including *Marathon: The Ultimate Training Guide,* now in its 4th edition, Higdon also has written books on many subjects and for different age groups. His children's book, *The Horse That Played Center Field,* was made into an animated feature by ABC-TV. He ran eight times in the Olympic Trials and won four World Masters Championships. One of the founders of the Road Runners Club of America (RRCA), Higdon also was a finalist in NASA's Journalist-in-Space program to ride the space shuttle. He has served as training consultant for the Chicago Marathon, hosts popular forums on Facebook and Twitter, and also offers online training programs through TrainingPeaks and apps through Bluefin. At the American Society of Journalists and Authors' annual meeting in 2003, the society gave Higdon its Career Achievement Award, the highest honor given to writer members. In its October 2015 issue, *Runner's World* included Higdon in its list of the 50 most influential people in running, ranking him first in a list of "gurus." An art major at Carleton College, he sells and exhibits his paintings in a Pop Art style. Hal Higdon's wife, Rose, hikes, bikes, skis, and supports him in his running and writing. They have three children and nine grandchildren.

Index

Underscored references indicate boxed text or tables.

F

G